NEW APPROACHES TO THE MANAGEMENT OF PRIMARY AND SECONDARY CNS TUMORS

Edited by **Lee Roy Morgan**

New Approaches to the Management of Primary and Secondary CNS Tumors
http://dx.doi.org/10.5772/63680
Edited by Lee Roy Morgan

Contributors

Serdar Altınay, Mihnea Zdrenghea, Delia Dima, Cristina Bagacean, Andrew Rodgers, Lee Roy Morgan, Ana Isabel Torres-Suárez, Juan Aparicio-Blanco, Marcus Ware, Michael Strong, Scott Turner, Mohammed Faraz Majeed, Muhammad Taimur Malik, Karolyn Au, Ying Meng, Suganth Suppiah, Anick Nater, Gelareh Zadeh, Rakesh Jalali, Michael Hayman, Jonathan Hayman

Published by InTech

Janeza Trdine 9, 51000 Rijeka, Croatia

Publishing Process Manager Iva Lipovic
Technical Editor SPi Global
Cover InTech Design team

First published March, 2017
Printed in Croatia
Legal deposit, Croatia: National and University Library in Zagreb

Additional hard copies can be obtained from orders@intechopen.com

New Approaches to the Management of Primary and Secondary CNS Tumors, Edited by Lee Roy Morgan
p. cm.
Print ISBN 978-953-51-3051-2
Online ISBN 978-953-51-3052-9

For EU product safety concerns:
IN TECH d.o.o., Prolaz Marije Krucifikse Kozulić 3, 51000 Rijeka, Croatia,
info@intechopen.com or visit our website at intechopen.com.

Meet the editor

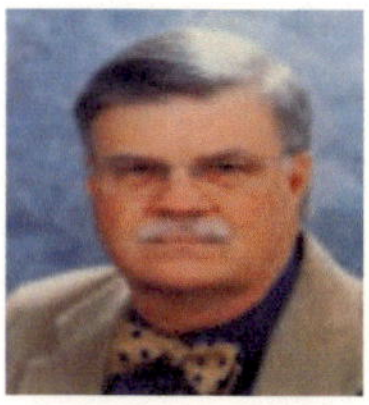

Dr. Lee Roy Morgan, MD, PhD, is a clinical pharmacologist and oncologist whose research interests are focused on the development of new and novel agents that penetrate the CNS and are effective against both primary and metastatic malignancies involving the CNS.

Dr. Lee Roy Morgan received his PhD degree in organic chemistry from Tulane University, New Orleans, Louisiana, in 1960. He completed his postdoctoral studies at Imperial College, University of London, in 1961. In 1971, he received his MD degree from Louisiana State University Medical School. From 1961 to 1986, he was a professor and the chairman of the Department of Pharmacology and Experimental Therapies, Louisiana State University Medical School, New Orleans, Louisiana, USA. He founded Dekk-Tec, Inc., in New Orleans, Louisiana in 1983 and is the CEO and director of research. In addition, he is an adjunct professor of Medicine in Tulane University School of Medicine and adjunct professor of Chemistry in the University of New Orleans, Louisiana. He has published over 200 research articles and book chapters. Dr. Morgan is married with four children and seven grandchildren.

Contents

Preface

The basic texture of research consists of dreams into which the threads of reasoning, measurements, calculations, and hard work are woven. The opportunity to edit *New Approaches to the Management of Primary and Secondary CNS Tumors* is an honor and privilege.

This book is dedicated to all students, researchers, health care professionals, and clinical investigators who have found delight in the serious contemplation of intellectual puzzles, promises, and rewards from neuro-oncology research and patient care. The gamut of interests in this book includes those of medicinal chemists, neurophysiologists, pharmacologists, laboratory scientists, and physicians. The chapters present reflections on the daily tasks of neuro-oncology researchers and health-care givers that include, but are not limited to, the design of new techniques, validating the best management care plans, and, in general, attempting to improve the health care for individuals with brain tumors.

Equally as important, the book includes the efforts of individuals who are contributing to the fundamental knowledge of the brain's biochemistry, physiology, chemistry, neurology, and biophysics, which are altered when cancer invades or develops in the brain and central nervous system.

The term chemobiodynamics is used in several chapters and represents the concept(s) by which the chemistry of a drug can manifest an impact on the hierarchy of molecular levels of living organisms. When cancer invades or develops in the central nervous system (CNS), there are major alterations in the normal hierarchy of cellular organization, which require different forms of cancer management (surgery, radiation, chemo-/immunotherapies, etc.). Unfortunately, therapies not only kill cancer cells but also damage normal tissues, including the immune system. Thus, the prefix "chemo" in chemobiodynamics could be replaced by immuno, neuro, radio, psycho, etc. with the same emphasis — to describe *effects that occur during the eradication of cancer involving the central nervous system.*

The present book attempts to review new approaches to the management of CNS tumors, and some chapters are presented that emphasize the development of novel chemical, radiological, and analytical techniques and therapeutics that can improve the care and management of subjects with neuro-oncological malignancies.

Since the book *Tumors of the Central Nervous System* (InTech) was published in 2014, neuro-oncology has made significant major progress; Phase I trials for new drugs have increased by 20-fold, and several drugs have been approved as target specific immuno-/chemotherapies for CNS malignancies. In addition, in the world of neuro-oncology, radiation therapy has radically evolved giving improved long-term survival and quality of life.

The authors that have written the chapters herein are “living their dreams and weaving their fibers" and are blessed. And, it is our wish that all of the readers are also able to pursue their dreams. Only through new concepts and endeavors are there any possibilities of converting cancers involving the brain and central nervous system into chronic illnesses followed by eradication.

Please continue to follow your dreams, because “Each of us has been chosen to accomplish our mission—we did not choose it!"

In summary, we have tried to bring together a wide range of interests and contributions from dozens of scientists and researchers to allow the readers to appreciate advancements in the management of neuro-oncology.

Lee Roy Morgan, MD, PhD
CEO
Dekk-Tec, Inc.
New Orleans, LA, USA

Section 1

Principles of Neuropharmacology

Chapter 1

NeuroPharmacology: As Applied to Designing New Chemotherapeutic Agents

Andrew H. Rodgers and Lee Roy Morgan

Additional information is available at the end of the chapter

http://dx.doi.org/10.5772/67591

Abstract

Neurooncology anticancer drugs are no exception—their distribution and tissue interactions follow the general rules of classical pharmacology. In an attempt to assist with the new therapeutic approaches to manage cancers involving the central nervous system, classical chemobiodynamic compartment and pharmacokinetic models are discussed and illustrated. In addition, strategies and approaches for penetrating the blood brain barrier (BBB) are reviewed and modeled. Finally, in support of classical pharmacology, a new anticancer agent in clinical trial for brain tumors is reviewed as an example of clinical onco-neuropharmacology.

Keywords: neurooncology, pharmacology, chemotherapeutics in clinical trials

1. Introduction

A basic assumption in cancer management is that all cancer cells must be killed or removed. When surgical and radiotherapies fail to achieve this goal, anticancer agents become the hope for control of the advanced disease.

Classically, when a drug is injected or orally administrated, ideally it is 100% absorbed and enters the systemic circulation and distributed into the various body compartments. The drug then develops equilibrium (distribution) between metabolism, storage, target tumors, nontumor organs, and final elimination [1].

The various body components and physiological barriers, which a cancer chemotherapeutic agent encounters from the time of administration until reaching the target site—the tumor—are depicted in **Figure 1** [2, 3].

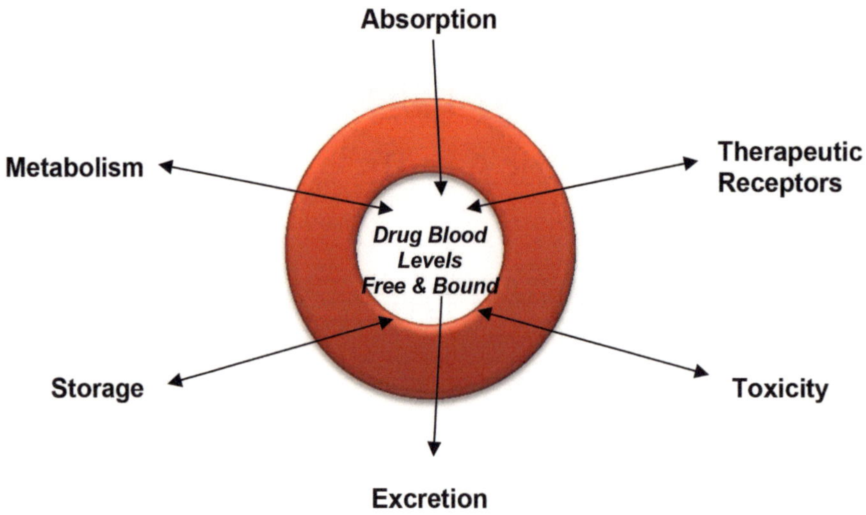

Figure 1. Drug distribution.

The intensity and duration of drug action at any one site depends upon absorption, distribution, affinity, excretion, and metabolism for the drug.

It is anticipated that the drug's tumor selectively will be such that it is absorbed preferentially, with relatively low toxicity to the host organs, such as bone marrow, liver, kidney, gastrointestinal tract, etc. In addition, the accumulation of drug in the tumor will depend upon lipid storage, metabolic activation, and elimination. The liver has a principal role in the metabolism of cancer chemotherapeutic agents, but the other organs such as bone marrow, liver, intestines, kidneys, and even brain also contain low levels of drug-metabolizing enzymes [1, 2].

Table 1 outlines the major types of biotransformation which anticancer drugs can be expected to undergo. These include oxidative, reductive, and conjugation reactions, which usually result in increased product polarity. The resulting product(s) are either activated or detoxified metabolites of the parent drug. The conjugated reactions usually result in water-soluble products, which are excreted *via* the biliary and urinary systems.

Oxidation reactions	Reductive reactions	Conjugation reactions
Aromatic hydroxylation	**1.** Keto reduction	**1.** Glucuronides
1. O^-, N^-, S^-, De-alkylation	**2.** Nitro reduction	**2.** Ethereal sulfates
2. Alkyl chain oxidation	**3.** Azo bond cleavage	**3.** Mercapturic acids
3. S-Oxidation		**4.** Amino acid conjugates
4. Oxidative deamination		**5.** Acetylated aromatic amines

Table 1. Biotransformation of drugs [4].

http://dx.doi.org/10.5772/67591

2. Cancer Cells Involving CNS

Cancer cells are the target of cancer chemotherapeutic agents, and the rate at which cancer cells interact with these agents is controlled by the hierarchy of molecular organization shown in **Figure 2**.

However, for tumor cells colonized in the brain and associated central nervous system structures, drugs/chemicals have an "additional hurdle," they must penetrate the blood brain barrier (BBB) before classical interactions and pharmacological principles can be applied. Evidence supports anticancer agents exerting their antitumor activities *via* cytotoxic, cytostatic and/or initiating immunotherapeutic mechanisms of action resulting in cancer cell death. All the chemotherapeutics interfere/interact with pathways in the cellular organization (**Figure 2**), thus inhibiting the synthesis of cancer cell DNA, RNA, proteins, and initiating lymphocyte—cancer cell recognition.

Although chemotherapeutics have their initial interactions on the molecular levels, they must first reach their targets. Thus, the abilities of chemotherapeutic agents to reach and interact with their targets are controlled by the hierarchy of distribution (**Figure 1**) and disposition (**Table 1**). These responses or changes are then transmitted to the respective molecular and/or cellular levels of cells (**Figure 2**).

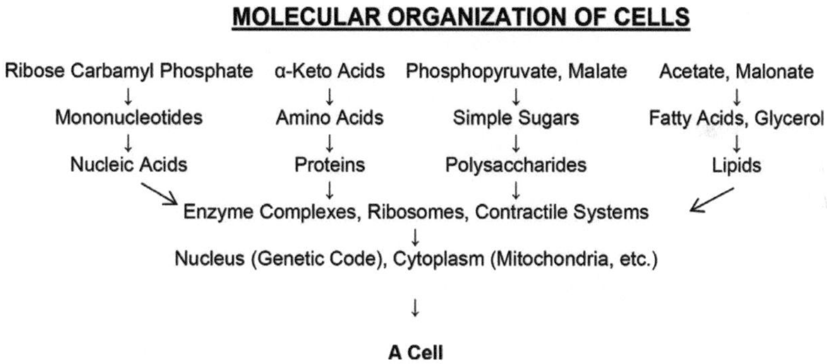

Figure 2. Hierarchy of cellular components. Molecular organization of cells.

3. Clark's correlates

In his classic work on general pharmacology, A.J. Clark divided the possible quantitative drug action(s) into five types [4]:

Relationship between:

(1) Time and the production of some quantitative response.

(2) Time and the incidence of some "all-or-none effect."

(3) Concentration and time of appearance of a selected action.

(4) Concentration and amount of quantitative response.

(5) Concentration and incidence of all-or-none effects.

The first three classes of Clark's correlates are expressions of kinetics and are the rate(s) of actions for drugs, while the last two classes summarize equilibrium conditions between drugs and their target sites. The reactivity of an agent with a molecular target in a biological system, is dependent upon the concentration of the "active therapeutic available" and often more important, is the rate at which the active form of the drug finds its way to the therapeutic sites/targets.

The selection of an optimal drug source requires consideration of:

(1) The qualitative and quantitative nature of the drug's known toxicity.

(2) The influence of drug concentration with time on tumor cell kill.

(3) The drug's pharmacology.

Consideration is also required for recovery time for the target organ, as well as nontarget organs, such as the bone marrow and gastrointestinal tract to recover prior to the administration of additional drugs. This depends on the pharmacologic disposition of the drug, since absorption, distribution, elimination, and metabolism affect the toxicity and efficacy, which can be achieved in the treatment of cancer.

4. Pharmacokinetics

Since most aspects of pharmacology involve dynamic processes, it is necessary to consider the rates or time courses for this process [5]. Pharmacokinetics is the quantitative measurement of concentration *vs.* time for drug and metabolite(s) in respective biological fluids, tissues, and for excretion. Pharmacokinetics is not the measurement of a solution to a problem; it is merely the scientific analysis of a drug's chemobiodynamics— the distribution of a drug in an organism [6].

Common questions in which applications of pharmacokinetics have proven to be useful include:

(1) How a drug is eliminated and how fast?

(2) What factors affect the rate of elimination?

(3) What is the optimal drug regimen for a drug?

(4) How can drugs and radiotherapy be combined?

(5) Is the pharmacological response due to the parent drug or a metabolite?

(6) Does drug distribution change with multiple dosing?

(7) How do the pharmacokinetics of chemically related drugs compare?

(8) How are the pharmacokinetics of a drug altered by the simultaneous administration of a second drug or radiation?

The initial step in a pharmacokinetic study is to determine if a drug is distributed by first or second-order reactions. The second step is to develop models for documentation.

4.1. First Order Kinetic Reactions

First-order reactions usually produce parallel curves for different doses of a drug with proportional shifts in the ordinate. If not, one must determine, which saturation processes or enzymatic reactions or zero order reactions are present.

Once the reaction kinetics is found to be first order, a model must be formulated. Models are based on the concepts of compartments. The simplest first order pharmacokinetics normally fits a one compartment model; for example, a drug is administered by intravenous injection and eliminated only in the urine or some other single route.

The rate of disappearance of the drug from the blood is proportional to the actual concentration of drug (x) in the blood (**Figure 3**).

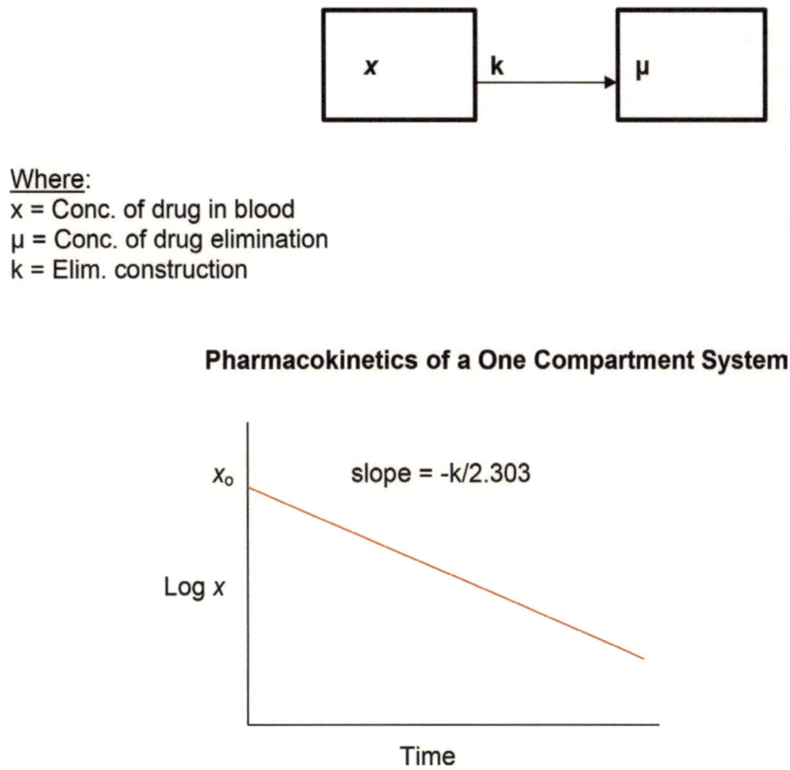

Figure 3. Pharmacokinetics of a one-compartment system.

Plotting the log [x] *vs*. time produces a slope equal to: −k/2.303.

The half-life ($t_{1/2}$) of the drug (x) is the time in which the concentration in the primary compartment decreases by 50%:

$$t_{1/2} = 0.693/\text{k}$$

The half-life is only meaningful as long as there is a one compartment model and the reaction is first-order. The half-life is also related to the clearance (*Cl*) and distribution (V_d) of the drug:

$$t_{1/2=}\, 0.693\; V_d/\text{Cl}, \quad \text{where } Cl = k \times V_d$$

and

$$V_{d=}\, \text{dose}/x_0\,; x_0 \text{ is obtained by extrapolating the curve to } t = 0.$$
$$\text{Also } -t_{1/2} = 06.93/\text{k} = 0.693\; V_d/Cl, \text{ where}: Cl = k\,V_d \text{ and } V_d = \text{dose}/x_0.$$

Thus, the elimination is calculated as – $dx/dt = -kx$ (with k = elimination constant)

4.2. Second Order Kinetic Reactions

Second-order reactions are best described in models where there are both elimination and distribution to other compartments and the curve would look like **Figure 4**. The upper portion of the curve represents distribution, while the lower flatter portion represents elimination [7].

The slope of the elimination phase or β is calculated by extending or extrapolating the lower portion of the curve to the ordinate (intercept) at B. The slope of the distribution phase or α is calculated by taking the differences between times for actual curve A and extrapolating to (B) back to T_0.

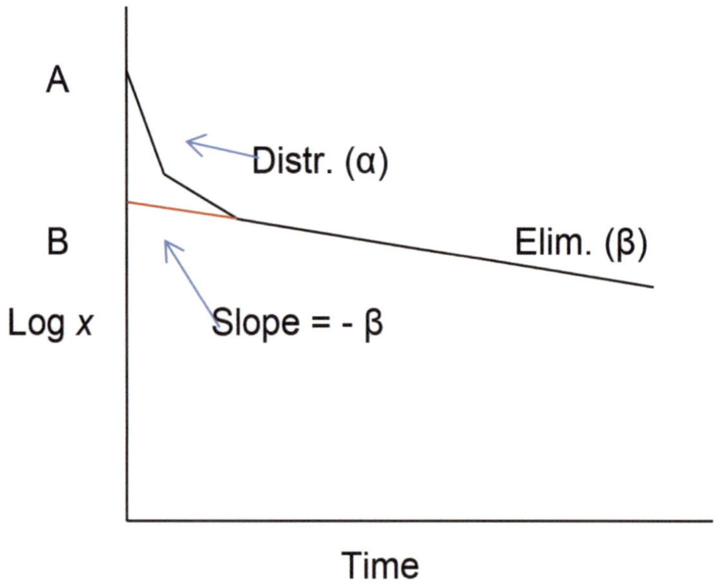

Figure 4. Pharmacokinetics of a two-compartment system [2].

http://dx.doi.org/10.5772/67591

Here, $t_{1/2}\ (\alpha) = 0.693/\alpha$ and $t_{1/2}\ (\beta) = 0.693/\beta$ – **Figure 4**.

There are some disadvantages to this type of feathering—data can be biased when converting from linear to log scale and objectivity lost (too much importance placed on the terminal part of the curve where there is often least confidence). Computer models are best employed, if possible.

In this type of example, it is meaningless to speak of $T_{1/2}$, since the whole curve is determined by two $T_{1/2}$ values analogous to K_1 and K_2, and one cannot combine these two values directly. It is no longer true that the $T_{1/2}$ values remain constant for greater than two compartments.

4.3. Drug Distribution

Another reason for the success or failure in drug activity is related to the pharmacologic disposition of drugs in subjects. Even if the tumor is sensitive to a drug, the latter is not useful unless it reaches the tumor site and remains there in cytotoxic (therapeutic) concentrations long enough to kill the tumor cells. In general, the purpose of pharmacology studies is to inform the treating physicians what is an effective concentration (*C*) of the drug that can be administered by a certain route and be present (available) for a sufficient period of time (*T*) to bring about the desired effect. This is referred to as the "optimal $C \times T$," and in most diseases, this can be approximated for dosing in humans through preclinical studies in animal models. Generally, 10% of the LD_{10} in mice is the acceptable starting dose [1].

4.4. Correlation of Pharmacokinetic Profile

What makes cancer different from other diseases is the need to relate optimal $C \times T$ to the phases of the cell cycle [1]. First, the optimal $C \times T$ for the tumor must be estimated for the real target—the tumor cells that are susceptible to be killed by the drug. Second, calculations are required to define the optimal $C \times T$ for human safety (e.g., the $C \times T$ that will be tolerated by normal organ tissues (bone marrow or gastrointestinal tract in most cases). Third, the cell population kinetics of both tumor cells and normal cells will be perturbed as a result of the drug's administration; however, the cancer cell growth fraction should be reduced to a greater degree, with sparing of normal tissues. Thus, the potential for drug's usefulness is a balance between anticancer activity and damage to healthy organs/tissues. Understanding the failure of active drugs to cause regression of cancer will depend to a significant extent upon successful delineation of this complex pharmacology.

Thus, the effectiveness of an antitumor agent is directly related to $C \times T$, which is markedly affected by dose, schedule, and its pharmacokinetics discussed above. The sensitivities of the cancer cells, as well as, normal tissue to drugs are the variable factors, which determine the potential usefulness of a drug. Documentation of the optimal $C \times T$ is usually conducted in Phase I studies and will relate clinical responses to acceptable doses and schedules necessary to standardize drug use in humans.

The optimum $C \times T$ should kill the maximum tumor cells with minimum lethality to cells of normal tissue.

The $C \times T$ product is also known as the area under the curve (AUC) and discussed and illustrated latter in this chapter.

5. Blood brain barrier

The chemobiodynamic relationship of a drug with the blood brain barrier (BBB) evaluated using *in vivo, in vitro,* and *in silico* (computational) models in attempt to appreciate the best design for novel anticancer agents to be used in subjects with malignant tumors involving the brain and central nervous system.

The blood brain barrier was discovered over 100 years ago by Paul Ehrlich who found that water soluble dyes stained all organs of animals except for their brains and central nervous system (CNS) [8]. Subsequently, other researchers found that Ehrlich's dye injected into the brain did not enter the blood stream and hence a barrier existed between the two compartments. These compartments could be traversed by more lipophilic substances however [9]. In general, more lipid soluble drugs can traverse the blood brain barrier by passive diffusion, while other molecules can cross the blood brain barrier (BBB) by active transport by proteins such as P-glycoprotein (P-gp) [10].

The BBB differs from normal capillaries in that it has tight junctions in the endothelial cell walls with specialized pores and junctions (formed by terminal surfaces of endothelial cells, neurons, astrocytes, etc.) that allow selective transport through the openings. The BBB is also highly electrically resistant confirming that it is very fatty and free of aqueous electrolytes [5].

To treat cancers involving the CNS, the BBB is the protective "no man's land" must be penetrated by anticancer agents. **Figure 5** depicts two modes of drug transport into the brain and intracerebral cancers. **Figure 5(a)** requires drug to penetrate *via* diffusion or a transfer pathway [12]. **Figure 5(b)** allows drugs to penetrate the CNS *via* the association with RBCs or transport through cancer-associated breaks in the BBB [11].

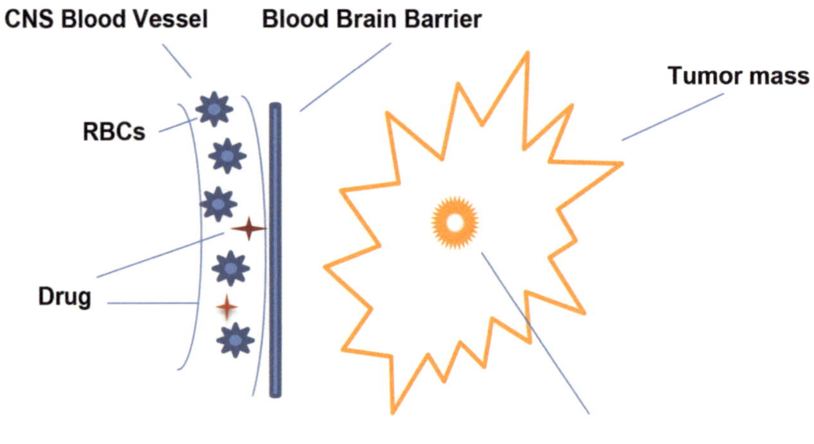

Figure 5a. Primary tumor mass involving the CNS. Drugs (+) can only penetrate the BBB by passive diffusion or active transport.

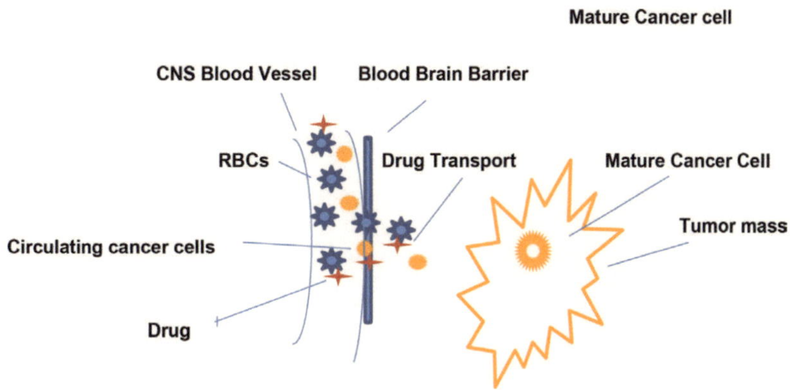

Figure 5b. Breaks (leaks) in the BBB 2° to cancer cell (●) penetration and tumor growth allow RBCs (✱) and associated drugs (+) easily penetration into tumors growing in the brain.

5.1. Calculation of Log *P*

Measuring or calculating log *P* is the most important molecular attribute to defining lipophilicity and the ability of the drug to diffuse across the lipophilic BBB. This is measured by dissolving the drug in octanol and then shaking with equal volumes of water. The concentration of drug is then measured in both phases and the ratio of octanol-water is calculated according to Eq. (1) [6].

$$\log P_{\text{octanol/water}} = \log\left([\text{solute}]_{\text{octanol}}/[\text{solute}]_{\text{water}}\right) \tag{1}$$

Since, very lipophilic compounds tend to be highly lipoprotein bound and associate/bind to lipid membranes, thus the ideal octanol-water partition coefficient for a neurotargeted drug (at pH 7.4) to diffuse from the serum into BBB into the CSF should be ≤ log *P* 5 [2, 12].

The estimation or determination of BBB permeability as $\log_{BBB}$ (the concentration of drug in the brain is divided by concentration in the blood) is accomplished as follows:

(1) *In vitro* kits to measure $\log_{BBB}$ in monkey or rat brain cells [13].

(2) *In vivo* during a clinical trial (Phase I).

(3) *In silico* computer models that simulate human BBB and are validated by correlating with drugs of known and measured $\log_{BBB}$ values [5]. For example, for DM-CHOC-PEN, temozolomide and others, log P can be calculated from their structure and from Eq. (2) $\log_{BBB}$ calculated [13–15].

$$\log_{BBB} = (\log P - 0/1725)/2.808. \tag{2}$$

Table 2 lists compounds with known brain and/or CNS activity and from their structure log *P* is calculated. From this value and Eq. (2) $\log_{BBB}$ is calculated; the latter is compared to literature values in **Table 2**. The calculated and literature values are in good agreement indicating that log *P* is a good predictor of passive diffusion through the BBB. However, one must realize

Compound	Structure	Calculated log P	Calculated $\log_{BBB}$	Calculated BBB	Actual BBB [15]
Cis-platinum	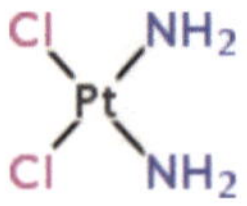	−2.83	−1	0.09	0.05–1
Cytarabine	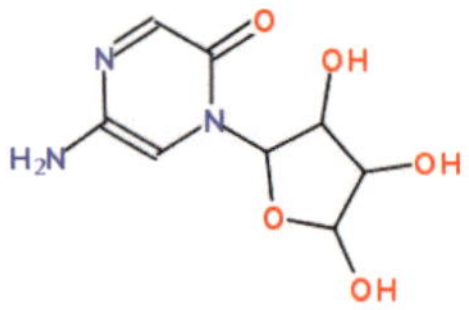	−2.77	−1	0.1	1
Pentostatin	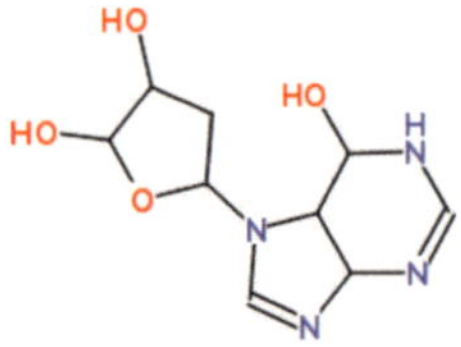	−2.35	−0.9	0.13	0.1-0.13
Temozolamide	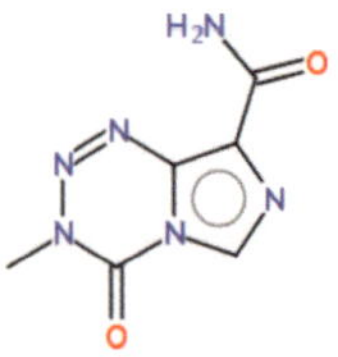	−1.9	−0.7	0.18	0.19
Cladribine	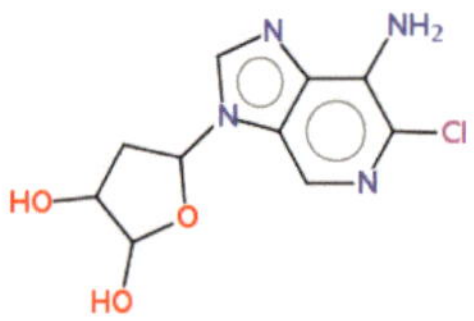	−0.38	−0.2	0.64	0.25
Dacarbazine	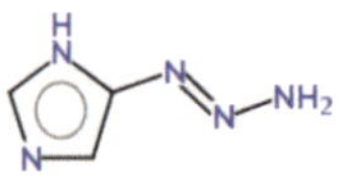	−0.35	−0.19	0.69	0.14
Melphalan	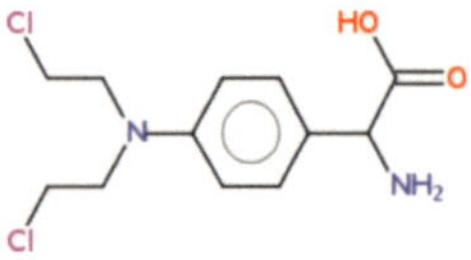	−0.01	−0.06	0.86	0.01–0.1
Busulfan	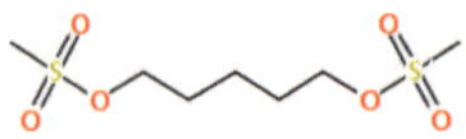	0.08	−0.03	0.9	1
Topotecan	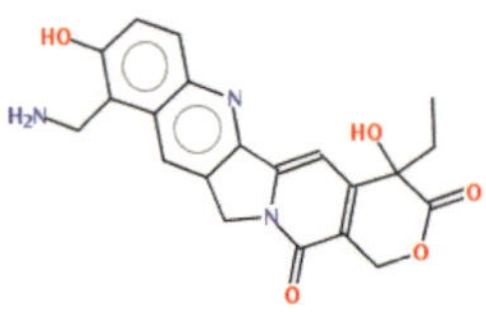	1.41	0.44	2.76	0.42
Carmustine	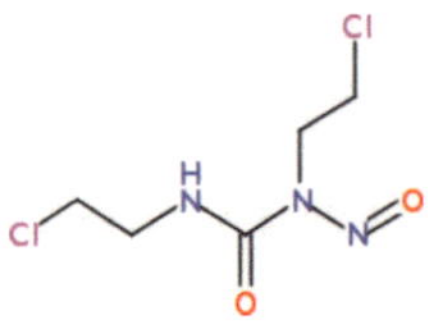	1.67	0.5	3.44	2.3–9

http://dx.doi.org/10.5772/67591

Compound	Structure	Calculated log *P*	Calculated $\log_{BBB}$	Calculated BBB	Actual BBB [15]
Lomustine	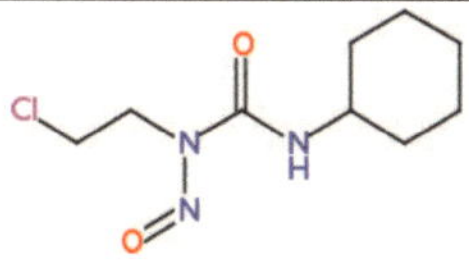	2.96	1	10	>0.5
DM-PEN	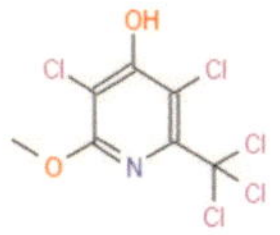	4.32	1.5	30	TBD
DM-CHOC-PEN	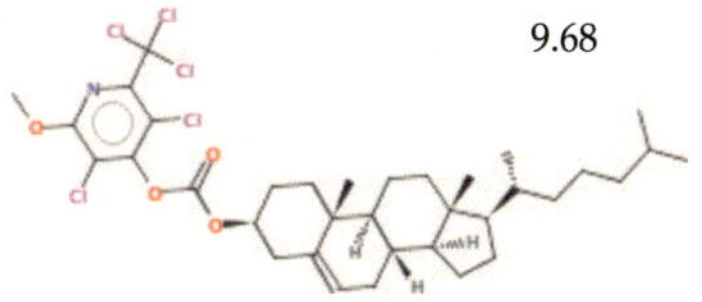	9.68	3.4	2431	TBD

Table 2. Calculated and structure related activities for molecules with known intracerebral activity [15].

that this is just a predictor of drug penetration across the BBB. Some drugs have higher cytotoxicity and selectivity than others and as such are active at lower concentrations than other drugs, e.g., temozolomide. Other caveats include the fact that drugs that penetrate the BBB can be "pumped out" — P-glycoprotein (GgP), thus the log *P* is not predictive that all drugs will be active [10, 15].

6. Clinical applications

The above introductory information provides the general principles, which must be considered when designing or planning on using a drug to treat cancer involving the brain.

4-Demethyl-4-cholesteryoxycarbonylpenclomedine (DM-CHOC-PEN) [**Figure 6**] is a lipophilic cholesterol carbonate polychlorinated pyridine that is cytotoxic and penetrates the BBB, both because of its $\log_{BBB}$ (**Table 2**), as well as an affinity for red blood cells (RBCs) [16–18].

6.1. DM-CHOC-PEN PK Profile With Cell Cycle

DM-CHOC-PEN's PK profile is best modeled *via* a two compartment model with ~5% being excreted unchanged in the urine [17]. The use of plasma pharmacokinetics is of great importance in considering its use. The drug has produced excellent responses in primary cancers (glioblastomas) as well as metastatic (lung, melanoma, breast) cancers involving the CNS [18]. DM-CHOC-PEN is lipophilic and penetrates the BBB, as well as transported and activated in metastatic cancers involving the CNS through a 4-tier mechanism: (1) transport per RBCs into the brain via breaks in the BBB; (2) entry into cancer cells per the L-glutamine (GLM) transfer system; (3) activation to DM-PEN (active molecule) *in situ* in the acidic microenvironment of cancer cells; and (4) *bis*-alkylation of DNA at N^7-guanine and N^4-cytosine—with cellular death [11].

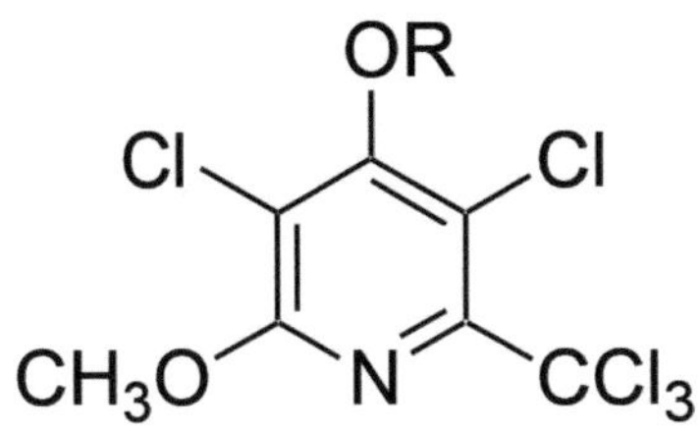

Where:

DM-CHOC-PEN: R=CO_2-cholesteryl

DM-PEN: R=H

Figure 6. DM-CHOC-PEN and metabolite DMPEN.

It's a large molecule and if there are liver metastases or other hepatic disease involving the liver there can be biliary congestion resulting in reversible jaundice [17].

The pharmacokinetics of DM-CHOC-PEN's disappearance from plasma after a single intravenous dose consist of an initial phase having a $T_{1/2}$ of 5 hours and a final phase $T_{1/2}$ of 245 hours (**Figures 7** and **12**). The slow, final phase of DM-CHOC-PEN elimination is the reason for the single high dose schedules that are currently being employed [18].

6.2. DM-CHOC-PEN Degradation

It has been found that the hydrolysis of DM-CHOC-PEN to DM-PEN (**Figure 7**) is the principle route of degradation and elimination of the drug in animals and humans [16].

Results vary with individual patients but on a mass balance analysis 1–10% of DM-CHOC-PEN are excreted unchanged and the metabolite, DM-PEN is excreted 10–100% in the urine. **Figure 8** shows a pattern seen for 12 subjects treated once with 70–85.8 mg/m^2 plasma and urine drug and metabolite levels [17].

6.3. Area under the curve

Increasing the dose of DM-CHOC-PEN increases the plasma concentration of drug and metabolites. The C_{max} increased with the dose giving rise to an increase in area under the curve (AUC) (**Figure 9**). **Figures 9** and **10** combine and summarize the AUCs for DM-CHOC-PEN *vs*. time [16, 17].

6.4. Distribution and elimination

DM-CHOC-PEN follows a standard two compartment model for elimination [17].

The preclinical and Phase I trial results suggest that the brain and central nervous system is targeted, but that all tissues including cancer tumors will absorb drug [17, 19]. So the second step in decreasing DM-CHOC-PEN blood levels is drug elimination. From bioavailability kinetic studies, this has found to be about 4%. The third step of elimination is after the metabolic degradation to a more water soluble and excreted as DM-CHOC-PEN. For DM-CHOC-PEN, the drug is primarily eliminated as DMPEN in the urine, which accounts for 57% of the dose on a mass balance basis. The metabolite on average has maximal plasma concentration 14 hours after drug administration (**Figure 8**) [17, 19].

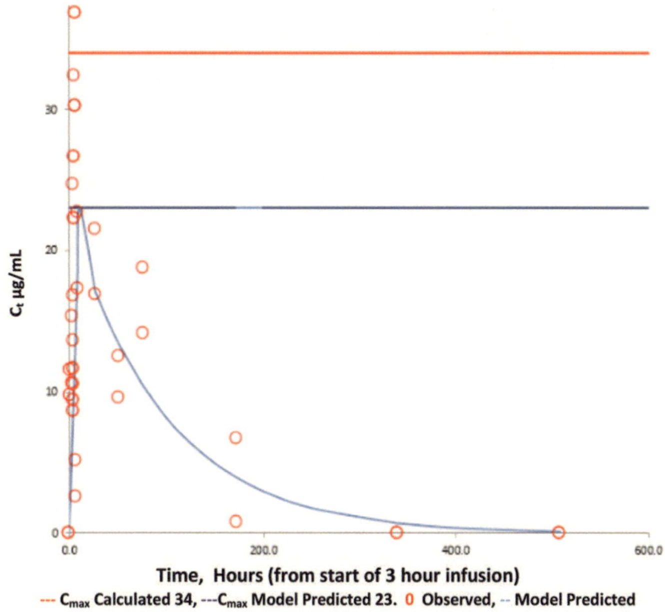

Figure 7. Plasma decay curve for DM-CHOC-PEN: 85.8 mg/m^2 IV once.

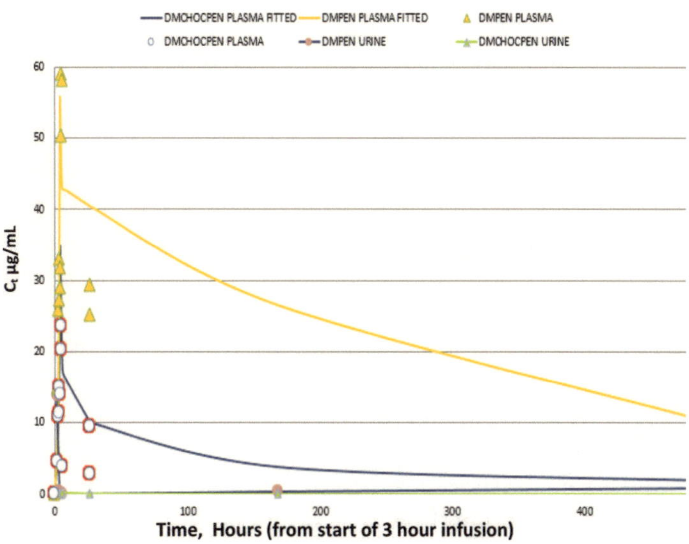

Figure 8. DM-CHOC-PEN + DM-PEN plasma and urine levels.

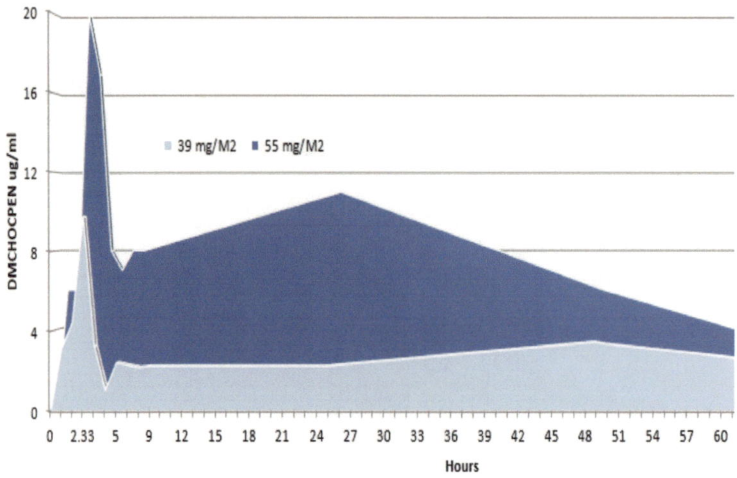

Figure 9. AUC—1 subject–doses of 39 mg/m², then 21 days later—55 mg/m².

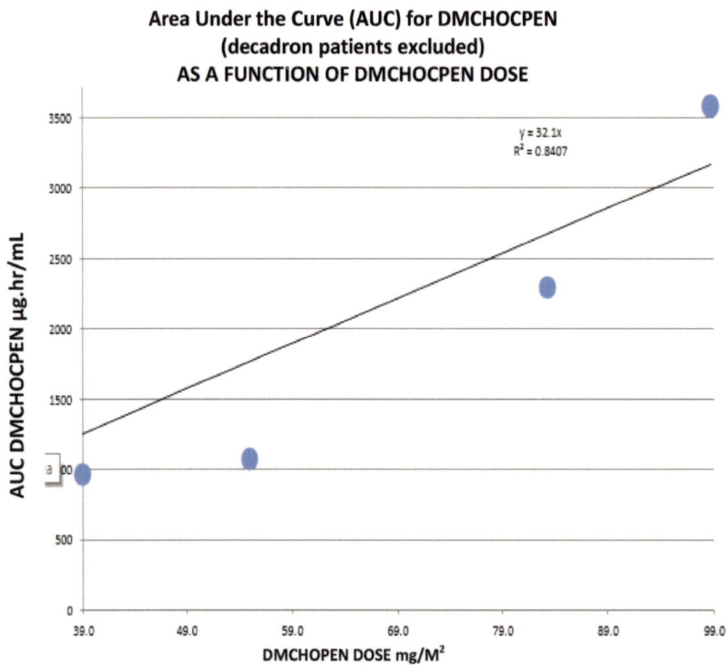

Figure 10. Area under the curve (AUC) for DMCHOCPEN (decadron patients excluded) as a function of DMCHOCPEN dose.

The whole point of the above discussion is to illustrate that there are differing kinetic processes involved in drug elimination such that elimination is not linear with time. In classical pharmacokinetics, this is described as two compartment model and you know you have one when you plot Log Drug Plasma Concentration *vs.* time and you see two slopes (**Figure 12**).

Thus, from the DM-CHOC-PEN and DM-PEN study, the drug is eliminated in a two compartment model (see **Figures 11** and **12**). In addition, DM-CHOC-PEN has been identified in the CNS and tumors as DNA adducts [17, 19].

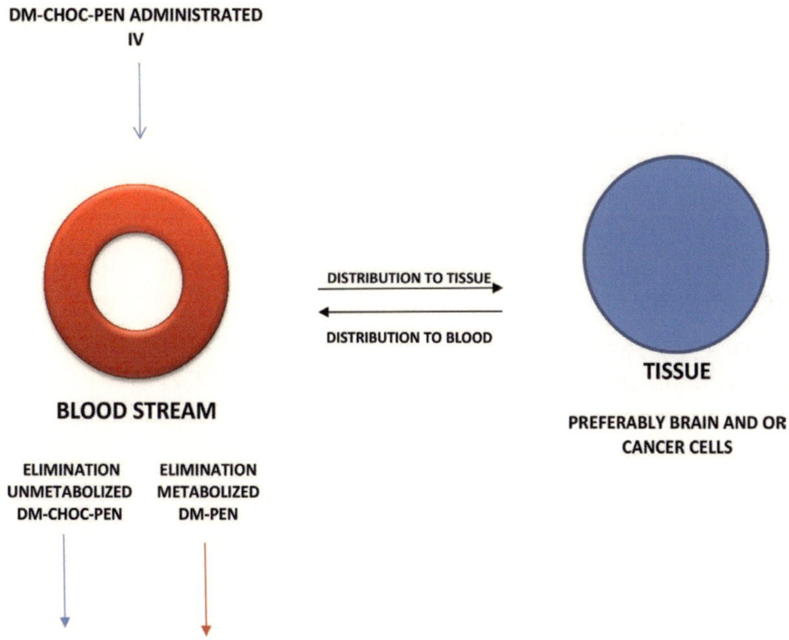

Figure 11. Distribution of DM-CHOC-PEN into the CNS and Cancer Cells.

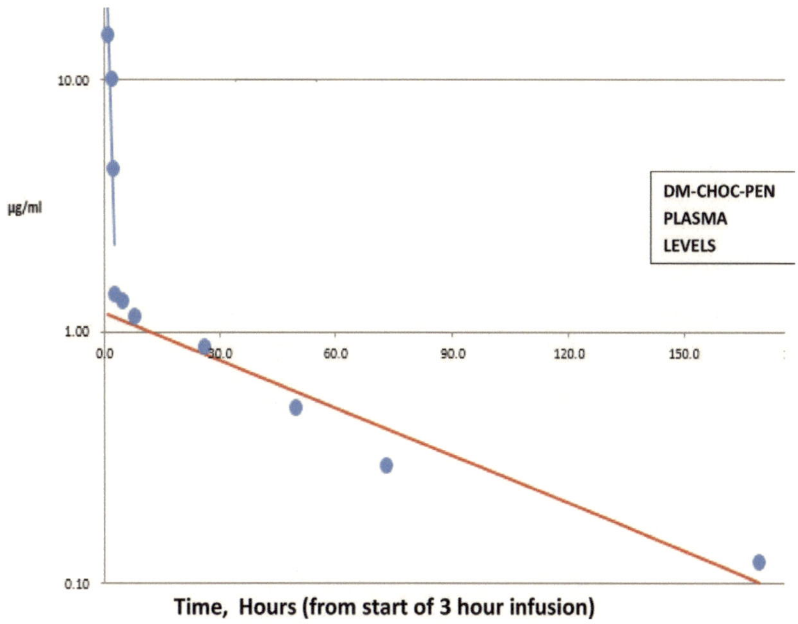

Figure 12. Elimination of DM-CHOC-PEN identified as two-compartment model as log plasma concentration *vs.* time is bi-linear two slopes evident initial α or distribution phase: terminal β or elimination phase.

7. Conclusion

An attempt to review neuropharmacology and distribution of anticancer agents in the central nervous system has been made. However, actually little is known about the interactions of drugs with the various levels of the CNS. We combined drugs in neurooncology but actually know little about the neuropharmacology of any single agent. In fact, Clark's basic pharmacological questions that should have been answered for all the agents we use but have been answered in only a few cases. With the current interests in neurooncology, we may finally make some progress in the specialty—but let's do it correctly.

Acknowledgements

Supported by NCI/SBIR grants – 5R44CA85021 and 3R43CA132257.

Author details

Andrew H. Rodgers* and Lee Roy Morgan

*Address all correspondence to: ahrodgers@gmail.com

DEKK-TECK, Inc. New Orleans, LA, USA

References

[1] Morgan, L.R., Principles of Pharmacology, Practical Oncology Today. Part II. Adra Labs, 1977.

[2] Morgan, L.R. and Weatherall, T.J., "*Pharmacology and drug distribution. In: Combined Modalities. Chemotherapy/Radiotherapy.*" Phillips, T.L. (ed.) Int. J. Radit. Oncol., Biol. Phys., 17, 20–24,1974.

[3] Oliverio, V.T. and Guarino, A.M., "*Absorption, protein binding, distribution, and excretion of antineoplastic drugs.*" Biochem. Pharmacol. 23, Supp 2:9–20, 1974.

[4] Clarke, A.J., General Pharmacology, in A. Heffter (ed.), "*Handbuch der experimentellen Pharmakologie,*" vol. 4, Springer-Verlag, Berlin, 1937, pp. 63–65.

[5] Goodman & Gilman's The Pharmacological Basis of Therapeutics, edition 11, Brunton, LL, Lazo, JS, Parker, KL, McGraw-Hill, New York, 2006,.

[6] Schuler, F.W., Chemobiodynamics and Drug Design, McGraw-Hill Book Co. New York, 1960.

[7] Germain, R., Bastian, G., Serota, D., Struck, R.F., Morgan, L.R., Isophosphoramide mustard (IPM): preclinical pharmacology and toxicology in rodents, dogs and primates. Cancer Chemother. Pharmacol., 51, 1204–1212, 2004.

[8] Ehrlich, P., Das Sauerstoff-Bedurfniss des Organismus. Eine farbenanalytische Studie. Verlag von August Hischwald 1–167, 1885.

[9] The Davis Lab. History of the Blood Brain Barrier, University of Arizona, Tucson, AZ 85721, 2014.

[10] Hartz, A.M.S. and Bauer, B., Regulation of ABC transporters at the blood brain barrier: new targets for CNS therapy. Mol. Interv., 10(5), 293–304, 2010.

[11] Morgan, L.R., Benes, E., Rodgers, A.H., Mahmood, T., Weiner, R.S., Cosgriff, T.S., Influence of L-Glutamine on DM-CHOC-PEN Activity in NSLC, 16th Int.Lung Cancer Congress, 2015.

[12] Carpenter, T.S., Kirshner, D.A., Lau, E.Y., Wong, S.E., Nilmeier, J.P., Lightstone, F.C., A method to predict blood brain barrier permeability of drug like compounds using molecular dynamic simulations. Index of compounds with data indicating they either cross or do not cross the BBB (or are found in CSF). Biophys. J., 107, 630–641, 2014.

[13] http://www.pharmacocell.co.jp/en/bbb/index_e.html

[14] http://www.molinspiration.com

[15] http://www.brynmawr.edu/chemistry/Chem/mnerzsto/bbb_index_of_compound-optimized.pdf

[16] Morgan, L.R., Struck, R.F., Rodgers, A.H., Jursic, B.S. Waud, W.R., Carbonate and carbamate derivatives of 4-demethylpenclomedine as novel anticancer agents. Cancer Chemother. Pharmacol., 64, 829–835, 2009.

[17] Weiner, R.S., Ware, M.L., Bastian, G., Rodgers, A.H., Urien, S., Morgan, L.R., Comparative pharmacokinetics of 4-demethyl-4-cholesteryloxycarbonylpenclomedine (DM-CHOC-PEN) in humans, Proc. Amer. Assoc. Cancer Res., 53, 758, 2012.

[18] Weiner, R.S., Friedlander, P., Gordon, C., Saenger, Y., Ware, R.L., Mahmood, T., Rodgers, A.H., Bastian, G., Urien, S., Morgan, L.R., Early clinical trial for 4-demethyl-4-cholesteryl-oxycarbonylpenclomedine (DM-CHOC-PEN) in patients with advanced cancer. Proc. Am. Assoc. Cancer Res., 56, 246, 2015.

[19] Morgan, L.R., Rodgers, A.H., Bastian, G., Benes, E., Waud, W.S., Papagiannis, C., Krietlow, D., Jursic, B.S., Struck, R.F., LaHoste, G., Thornton, M., Luttrell, M., Stevens, E., Thompson, R., Comparative preclinical pharmacology and toxicology for 4-demethyl-4-cholestryloxylcarbonylpenclomedine (DM-CHOC-PEN) – a potential neuro-alkylating agent for glioblastoma (GBM) and metastatic cancers involving the central nervous system. *In*: Morgan, LR (ed.): Tumors of the Central Nervous System – Primary and Secondary, Rijeka, InTech; 2014, pp. 239–263.

Section 2

Diagnosis of CNS Tumors

Chapter 2

Role of Pathologist in Driver of Treatment of CNS Tumors

Serdar Altınay

Additional information is available at the end of the chapter

http://dx.doi.org/10.5772/65911

Abstract

The incidence of Central Nervous System (CNS) tumors is gradually increasing. Furthermore, metastatic neoplasms are frequently seen in neuropathology practice as a major cause of mortality and morbidity. Pathologists try to reach a more accurate diagnosis by mentally filtering a synthesis, comprising age, radiological characteristics and microscopic findings in the sample sent, starting already from the intraoperative diagnosis process. By displaying their skills, they unveil whether a lesion in the brain parenchyma is a normal or reactive tumor and if this is a tumor, is it primary or metastatic, and if it is primary, what is the tumor type or if it is metastatic, which organ could it be associated with. Pathologists use diagnostic, prognostic and predictive markers in order to enable the patient receive the most effective and sufficient treatment. They ensure that an individualized treatment is provided via these tools, by making a histological diagnosis of the lesion according to the WHO classification, identifying the course of the disease and preventing undesired and dangerous complications. This chapter will focus on answering these questions and share the value of a multidisciplinary approach in the management of brain tumors in neurosciences, which is gradually increasing in importance, and how pathologists execute this art.

Keywords: pathology, central nervous system, primary or metastatic tumor, neuropathology, oncologic treatment

1. Introduction

Brain tumors could be classified according to the histogenesis and microscopic similarities of the tumors in the previous decades, and their degree of differentiation was identified. This characterization was a simulation effort of pathologists via the utilization of light microscopy, immunohistochemical markers and ultrastructural methods [1–3].

There were two major concepts accepted as basis in the WHO classification: the histological type and histological degree of the tumor.

Histological typing of the tumor: Histological typing in the WHO system was performed by defining the entity, variant and tissue pattern characteristics. The tumor group, which constituted clinicopathological integrity, where the cellular origin or the cell type from which they derived was accepted as common and formed the subtitles of the relevant section in the WHO booklet, was named entity; the tumor group, which belonged to an entity, was a tumor type of an original character from a clinical, morphological and/or molecular aspect and formed the subtitles of the relevant section in the WHO booklet, which was named a variant; and the tumor group, which had an original morphological character, did not differ from the other tumors of the entity from a clinical, molecular and/or prognostic sense and generally formed the paragraph titles of the section on entity, which was named tissue pattern.

WHO	Features of Grading
Grade I	have low proliferative potential and able to cure with surgical resection
Grade II	usually have diffuse infiltrative and low proliferative potential, but probability of low recurrence rate, some of them have risk of progression to high grade
Grade III	mostly known as anaplastic tumors and have malign histologic features, have high recurrence rate, usually need chemotherapy and radiotherapy
Grade IV	obviously malign tumors, which are necrotic and have capability of fast recurrence, most of them show diffuse spreading in CNS

Table 1. Characterization of CNS tumors according to the WHO grading.

Tumor grading: Grade IV was assigned for CNS tumors in relation to the cytological and histological criteria of WHO (WHO Grade I–IV) (**Table 1**). These grades were based on histopathological criteria fundamentally characterizing malignancies and also comprised the prediction of the clinical course of the patient [4].

The classification and grading system was a universally accepted and mostly easily repeatable system. However, there were some points which were not substantiated with sufficient data and posed problems in terms of repeatability within this system; 2007 classification was prepared by more than 70 specialists, in light of the literature data obtained until that time. The studies conducted on brain tumors in the last two decades unveiled the genetic basis of

http://dx.doi.org/10.5772/65911

tumorogenesis and demonstrated that it is possible to contribute to the classification of these tumors [5–11]. In fact, the Haarlem meeting held in 2014 paved the way for a major revision in the 2007 CNS classification of incompatible molecular findings in the diagnosis of brain tumors [12]; 2016 CNS WHO classification was prepared with the contribution of 117 participants from 20 countries and 35 neuropathologists and neuro-oncologists from 10 countries who elaborated on topics of debate [13].

This chapter will focus on active immunohistochemical evaluation in the diagnostic approach toward primary tumors and tumors with unknown primary, how to conduct differential diagnostics on metastatic tumors and the major changes in the current CNS tumor classification and will briefly describe the role undertaken by pathologists in guiding the treatment of CNS tumors.

2. Incidence of brain tumors and overview

The annual incidences of central nervous system tumors correspond to 10–17 in 100 thousand persons for intracranial tumors and 1–2 in 100 thousand persons for intraspinal tumors. Approximately half or three-fourth of these are primary tumors, while the rest are metastatic [14–16].

Central Brain Tumor Registry of the United States (CBRTUS), a professional research organization in the United States, which provides high-quality statistical data, recently published its report covering the years 2008–2012 [17]. Hence, malignant brain and CNS tumors constitute the 11th most prevalent types of cancer and the 3rd most frequent cause of mortality due to cancer in adolescents and young adults (AYAs). The most frequently diagnosed histologies in the AYA group are variable both in children (0–14 years) and in older adults (40+ years). While 53,083 adolescents and young adults (aged 15–39 years) in the United States were diagnosed with primary brain and CNS tumor between 2008 and 2012, the annual incidence rate was lowest in New England (9.42 per a population of 100,000) and the Pacific region (9.47 per a population of 100,000), and it was highest in the Middle Atlantic region (11.66 per a population of 100,000) and the Mountain region (11.14 per a population of 100,000). Knowing the age-specific histology of brain tumors and providing accurate statistical data enable clinicians to treat patients and provide reference to investigators for investigating new therapeutic agents.

Tumors in the central nervous system hold a larger share among childhood cancers and constitute almost 20% of all tumors. Childhood central nervous system tumors differ from the tumors in adults in terms of both their histological subtypes and location. Childhood tumors mostly tend to develop in the posterior fossa, while adult tumors are mostly seen in the supratentorial region [14–18].

The tumors in the nervous system bear specific characteristics which distinguish them from the neoplastic processes localized in the other regions of the body.

- A premalignant or in situ period is not identified in these tumors as in carcinomas.

- While even the most malignant gliomas rarely spread outside the CNS, the subarachnoid space allows tumor diffusion to distant regions along the neural axis, in addition to local infiltration [9, 14].

2.1. Practical use of immunohistochemistry in the diagnosis of CNS tumors

IHC has been undergoing a revolutionary process with an increasing use in diagnostic pathology in the last 50 years [19, 20]. While pathologists would say "insufficient biopsy for diagnosis" when they saw notably marked artifact areas in tiny biopsies in the past, today carcinoma diagnosis can be easily made with the cytokeratin (CK) stain [21]. If used wisely and combined with morphological interpretation skills, pathologists may achieve a more accurate diagnosis than "suspicion of malignancy." Thus, IHC markers may be divided into three as those used for diagnostic purposes, those used for prognostic purposes and the other IHC markers (**Table 2**).

IHC markers used for diagnostic purpose
Markers for glial tumors
GFAP
S-100
Markers for neuronal tumors
Synaptophysin
NSE
Beta-tubulin
Neurofilament
MAP-2
GFAP +/−
Markers for meningeal tumors
EMA
Vimentin
S-100
CK
Markers for choroid plexus tumors
CK
S-100
Transthyretin
Markers for lymphoma
LCA
T cell and B cell markers
Markers for Schwann cell tumors
S-100
Leu 7

http://dx.doi.org/10.5772/65911

IHC markers used for diagnostic purpose
Markers for germ cell tumors
AFP
HCG
PLAP
HPL
Markers for melanocytic tumors
HMB-45
S-100
MART-1 (Melan-A)
Microphthalmia transcription factor
Markers for vascular origin tumors
CD34
Factor VIII
VEGF
Ulex europaeus
Markers for pituitary tumors
PRL
GH
ACTH
MSH
LH
FSH
TSH
Markers for neuroendocrine tumor
Chromogranin
Synaptophysin
Marker for ATRT
INI-1/SMARCB-1
IC markers used for prognostic purpose
Cell cycle/proliferation markers
MIB-1
Ki-67
PCNA
BrdU
Tumor suppressor gene/oncogene protein
p53 tumor suppressor gene
Retinoblastoma tumor suppressor gene (Rb)
C-myc oncogene
Growth factors/receptors

IHC markers used for diagnostic purpose
EGFR
The IHC markers
IDH1 and IDH2
ATRX
BRAF

GFAP, glial fibrillary acidic protein; IHC, immunohistochemistry; CK, cytokeratin; NSE, neuron-specific enolase; MAP-2, microtubule-associated protein-2; EMA, epithelial membrane antigen; LCA, leukocyte common antigen; AFP, alpha fetoprotein; HCG, human chorionic gonadotropin; PLAP, placental alkaline phosphatase; HPL, human placental lactogen; HMB-45, human melanoma black-45; VEGF, vascular endothelial growth factor; PRL, prolactin; GH, growth hormone; ACTH, adrenocorticotrophic hormone; MSH, melanocyte-stimulating hormone; LH, luteinizing hormone; FSH, follicle stimulating hormone; TSH, thyroid stimulating hormone; ATRT, atypical teratoid/rhabdoid tumor; MIB-1, molecular immunology Borstel-1; Ki-67, Kiel antibody-67; PCNA, proliferating cell nuclear antigen; BrdU, bromodeoxyuridine; EGFR, epidermal growth factor receptor; IDH1 and IDH2, isocitrate dehydrogenase-1 and -2; ATRX, alpha-thalassemia/mental retardation syndrome X-linked.

Table 2. Immunohistochemistry markers for central nervous system tumors [21].

Despite being a highly beneficial diagnostic tool, the limitations of IHC should also be recognized. The amount of antigen in tumors is variable. As the antigenic phenotype of tumor cells is measured with IHC, its antibody immune activity is nonspecific. Furthermore, the high number of markers used for a tumor raises the cost. Therefore, pathologists should pay attention to the compliance with tumor morphology and the clinical-radiological correlation when interpreting the outcome of an IHC. Immunohistochemical markers may be used within the framework of differential diagnosis in surgical neuropathology.

Astrocytoma, oligodendroglioma or mixed tumors? Currently, there is still no agreement reached among specialists regarding this topic, and the most experienced specialists cannot reach an agreement on this topic. The following table reflects one of the approaches to this topic and was prepared in light of current data [22–24]. Glial, glioneural or reactive? Some of the cells seen in many tumors are the normal residual cells as residues of the tissue occupied by the tumor following tumor infiltration. Neuronal cells which may be seen inside diffuse astrocytoma constitute the most typical example. We should also add the question of whether the lesion is reactive or neoplastic to this differential diagnosis [24, 25]. Glial vs glionöronal tumors: GFAP, Olig-2, synaptophisin, Neu-N, neurofilament protein, p53, isocitrate dehydrogenase 1 (IDH1), CD34, BRAF v600e antibodies. Glial tumors vs gliosis IDH1, Ki67, p53, WT-1, CD68, LCA, GFAP, EGFRvIII antibodies. Glial tumors vs demyelinisian diseases: IDH1, p53, Olig-2, CD68, GFAP, JC virus, myelin basic protein and neurofilament antibodies. Mesenchymal tumor, but which one? The first series of findings to determine the panel to be selected in the differential diagnosis of mesenchymal tumors are clinical and radiological data. In particular, the localization of the tumor determines the tumor types included into the bounds of possibility. It is very difficult to establish a panel series comprising each possibility in this topic. The panels which may be used according to localization have been provided below only as recommendation [26–28].

Schwannoma vs meningioma: S100, neurofilament, Sox2, EMA, progesterone receptor, collagen type IV, CD34 antibodies. Meningioma vs solitary fibrous tumor: EMA, progesterone receptor, CD34, collagen type IV, bcl2, CD99 antibodies. Chordoma vs chondrosarcoma: Brachyury, S100, vimentin, cytokeratin cocktail and EMA antibodies.

2.2. Neuroradiological tips for pathologists in surgical neuropathology

The concepts associated with localization are among the major concepts in neuroradiology. Assessments from various planes are made: the sagittal (vertical) section analyzes the brain as right and left, the coronal plane analyzes it as frontal and back, and the axial (horizontal) plane assesses its upper and lower parts. Moreover, the main modalities in anatomic imaging are the contrast images obtained by administering T1, T2, FLAIR and gadolinium. In addition to these four modalities, also diffusion, perfusion and spectroscopic methods provide valuable insight into MR imaging [29].

MR imaging is composed of tones of gray between black and white, as in CT. The tissues which receive an energy signal equivalent to that of the brain tissue in the brain MRI and are thus seen as at the same tone of gray are defined as "isointense"; those which receive more signal and appear whiter are named "hyper-intense," while those which receive less signal and appear darker gray are defined as "hypo-intense." It is possible to obtain different sequences at different images by modifying some shooting parameters in the MRI imaging. Basically, we may list the MRI sequences as *T1-weighted, proton-intense and T2-weighted*. In T1-weighted images, the cerebrospinal fluid (CSF) appears black; in proton-intense images, it appears gray; and in T2-weighted images, it appears white. The lesions are generally "hyper-intense" in proton-intense and T2-weighted sequences, while they are "hypo-intense" in T1-weighted sequences. In addition to the basic sequences, there also other sequences which suppress the cerebrospinal fluid and enable fluids to appear hypo-intense (such as fluid attenuated inversion recovery—FLAIR) [29, 30].

Unlike CT, a paramagnetic contrast agent containing gadolinium is used in MRI. Gadolinium has a much lower risk to cause allergic reactions compared to iodine contrast agents. Gadolinium permeates to pathological tissues with a destroyed blood-brain barrier as in iodine contrast agents. Only T1-weighted sequences are applied after administering gadolinium. The lesions involving the contrast agent gain a hyper-intense appearance in T1-weighted MRI appearances. The tumor lesions other than low-degree glial tumors, metastatic tumors, infections (meningitis and encephalitis), demyelinating lesions during the acute period and infarcts during the subacute period demonstrate contrast agent involvement. When the lesion has a contrast agent involvement, it may be used in the differential diagnosis of the lesion and also in defining the degree of the lesion in primary brain tumors. Generally, the tumors with contrast agent involvement have a high-degree histopathology. (There are some exceptions to this generalization. For instance, although pilocytic astrocytoma is a low-grade glial tumor, it has a considerably high contrast agent uptake.)

It is possible to analyze the chemical content of tissues with the *MR spectroscopy (MRS)*, which is another MR imaging technique. *N-acetyl aspartate (NAA), creatinine (Cr), choline (Cho)* and *myo-inositol (mI) are major neurometabolites which may be detected via* MR spectroscopy. NAA is accepted as a neuro-axonal marker in the MRS assessment. It is known that neuro-axonal function is directly proportional to the number and concentration of NAA. Myo-inositol is used as an astrocyte marker. Pathologies which lead to an increase in the number of astrocytes inside the tissue (such as astrocytoma, encephalitis and subacute-chronic demyelinating plaques) elevate the myo-inositol concentration at MRS. Choline is a neurometabolite present on the cellular membrane and the myelin structure. Therefore, pathologies which lead to cellular proliferation (neoplastic diseases) or myelin destruction (demyelinating diseases) give rise to a notable increase in the choline level [29–32].

Infrared (IR) spectroscopic image system, which is a new method, is promising in identifying the primary in brain metastases. As metastatic cells comprise molecular information on the primary tissue and the probes of IR spectroscopy are the fingerprint of cells, this method introduces a new approximation method to the origin of brain metastases [31, 32].

2.3. Molecular pathological assessment in glial tumors

Molecular studies started with the identification of various clinical behaviors of oligodendroglial cells with 1p19q co-deletion. The detection of three major signal pathways [TRK/RAS/P1 (3) K (88%), P53 (87%) and Rb (78%)] initiated a new era in neuro-oncology [22, 33, 34].

The analysis of the number of DNA copies provided a new perspective in the evaluation of the gene expression profiles and the actual roles of the DNA methylation patterns and ERBB2, NF1 and TP53 genes. It unveiled the clinical and fundamental importance of the promotor methylation of MGMT genes. Today, it is accepted that treated glioblastoma (GBM) cases reveal the phenotype associated with the mismatch repair deficiency [35–37].

These developments demonstrated that the WHO 2007 CNS classification needs to be updated. It is necessary to include molecular data into the classification and to utilize the most appropriate, most widespread and convenient techniques in order to detect these. Thus, the Haarlem meeting was held in order to determine the usability of current diagnostic methods upon taking into account the clinical, experimental and etiological chance of correlation in the future and also considering the cost, without disrupting the current clinical and patient approach, and a consensus was reached. An integrated diagnosis comprises the histological diagnosis + WHO grading (histological grading) + molecular information or the Haarlem "layered diagnosis format" [12] (**Figure 1**).

Parsons et al. [37] published the (amplification and/or deletion) patterns of the protein coding 20.661 gene in human GBMs. New methodologies (aCGH, high-density oligonucleotide arrays, next-generation sequencing technologies, single nucleotide genomics, massively parallel DNA resequencing) confirmed the most unexpected results of the authors. The earliest genetic modification in most glial tumors impacts the gene which encodes the active area of the cytoplasmic form of a carbohydrate metabolizing enzyme (e.g., IDH, isocitrate dehydrogenase). Although there are many isoforms of this enzyme, the accepted IDH1 mutations are most prevalent in secondary GBMs occurring in relatively young patients with a better prognosis. These results were confirmed also by Balss et al. [38] and Yan et al. [39], and it was demonstrated that IDH mutations emerge in the systemic forms of rather specific and malignant diseases of glial tumors. Zhao et al. [40] published their observations in 2009 and showed that the mutations (IDH1 R132 or IDH2 R172) reduce the affinity of the enzyme toward the substrate and, moreover, inactive heterodimers which dominantly block the WT-IDH1 activity. The rapid understanding of the molecular pathways of the pathogenesis of brain tumors especially in glial tumors led to the detection of reliable diagnostic, prognostic and predictive molecular markers and new molecular signatures [41].

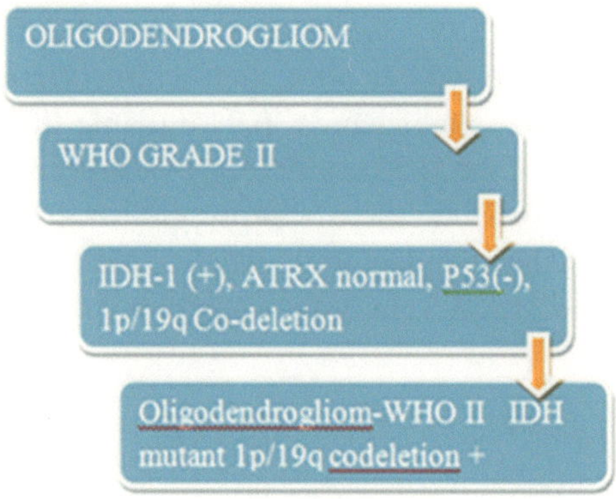

Figure 1. An example of integrated diagnosis according to the Haarlem consensus.

Three molecular markers, namely 1p19q co-deletion, MGMT promoter methylation mutation and mutation in IDH1/2 genes, stand out in the management of disease course and surgical neuropathology routine at the basis of various clinical trials.

Simultaneous loss of 1p/19q in glial tumors: It was demonstrated that chromosomes 1p and 19q are characterized with combined allelic deletion in 80% of oligodendroglioma (Grade II), 60% of anaplastic oligodendroglioma (Grade III) and 50% of mixed glioma [42, 43]. Two clinical studies demonstrated that in case of combined 1p/19q loss in the tumor bed, anaplastic glioma patients benefit from combined radiotherapy + PCV chemotherapy [44, 45]

MGMT promoter methylation: As a DNA repair enzyme, O6-methylguanine DNA methyltransferase (MGMT) reuptakes the alkylation of the O6 position of guanine, thus leading to apoptosis. MGMT promoter methylation results in the silencing of the gene in relation to the increase in the insufficiency of the DNA damage repair and reduces DNA repair damage with alkali chemotherapeutic agents such as temozolamide. MGMT promoter methylation appears in 40% of primary glioblastomas (WHO Grade IV) and is associated with the increase in life expectancy following radiotherapy and temozolamide chemotherapy [46, 47].

IDH1 and IDH2 mutations: IDH (isocitrate dehydrogenase) and its mitochondrial isoform IDH2 encode the protein catalyzing isocitrate to α-ketoglutarate and play an important role in the cellular control of this oxidative process. IDH1/2 mutations globally result in the functional changes of the tumor epigenome. The presence of somatic IDH1/2 point mutations is helpful in the differentiation of primary glioblastomas in most low-grade gliomas and secondary glioblastomas and the differentiation of pilocytic astrocytoma and the other brain tumors characterized with this mutation. The presence of IDH1/2 mutations in anaplastic gliomas and glioblastomas also has a prognostic significance as IDH-mutant tumors have a longer overall survival compared to IDH wild-type neoplasms [48]. Certainly, continuous definition of new molecular markers widens the diagnostic molecular spectrum of brain tumors and strengthens the art of neuropathology.

2.4. Problematic tumors in grading and major changes in 2016 CNS WHO

The major arrangement in WHO 2016 classification involved diffuse gliomas, medulloblastomas and other embryonal tumors. They were divided into three groups, namely glioblastoma, glioblastoma wild type, glioblastoma IDH-mutant, diffuse midline glioma and H3K27M-mutant, and the use of the NOS terminology was recommended when the molecular tests were not carried out or when there was no problem [13] (**Table 3**). Medulloblastomas were divided into widely accepted four genetic (molecular) groups, namely WNT-activated, SHH-activated and group 3 and group 4, which did not reveal either of these and were defined numerically.

*Glioblastom, IDH-wild type (**entity**)	
Giant cell glioblastom Gliosarcom Epithelioid glioblastom (**new variant**)	**variant**
<u>*Subtypes*</u>	
Smal cell glioblastoma Glioblastoma with primitive neuronal component Granuler cell glioblastoma Containing lipid or lipidise glioblastoma	**patern**
*Glioblastoma IDH mutant (**entity**)	
*Diffuse midline glioma, H3 K27M-mutant (**entity**)	
*Glioblastoma NOS	

Table 3. Classification of glioblastomas according to the WHO CNS 2016.

GBM with PNET components was a largely accepted subgroup and was designated as a pattern in 2016. Very distinct and small cell focal tumor nodules are present in the glioblastomas with PNET components. Neuronal differentiation differs compared to other fields. Furthermore, there is also the possibility to find MYC gene amplification in fields similar to PNET. However, the difference in prognosis, claimed to be present between variants and patterns, has not be proven yet. Although it is not certain whether there are differences between GBM with oligodendroglioma components and anaplastic oligodendrogliomas, some points which may be helpful for pathologists are summarized below.

Giant cell glioblastoma is a tumor with generally superficial localization, mostly composed of pleomorphic cells with scattered giant cells in between them. The most important point in differential diagnosis is that pleomorphic xanthoastrocytomas with anaplastic characteristics are not confused with this tumor.

Small cell glioblastoma is a monotonous tumor with a high number of mitosis, which may be confused with anaplastic oligodendrogliomas. Generally, it does not involve a 1p19q deletion and comprises EGFR gene amplification or mutant (EGFRvIII) forms [13, 37].

Glioblastomas with oligodendroglioma components constitute one of the most debated subtypes. This tumor may comprise fields in the typical oligodendroglial morphology, in addition to the classical glioblastomas and components including two different anomalies in some cases. The diagnosis is accepted as anaplastic oligodendroglioma in patients who previously have low-grade oligodendroglioma.

A chordoid glioma case of the third ventricle, which did not show such a high MIB-1 index (**Figure 2**) so far, was presented recently [49]. Interestingly, this patient had a long survival period. These cases will enter into the WHO CNS classification maybe as atypical chordoid glioma in the future.

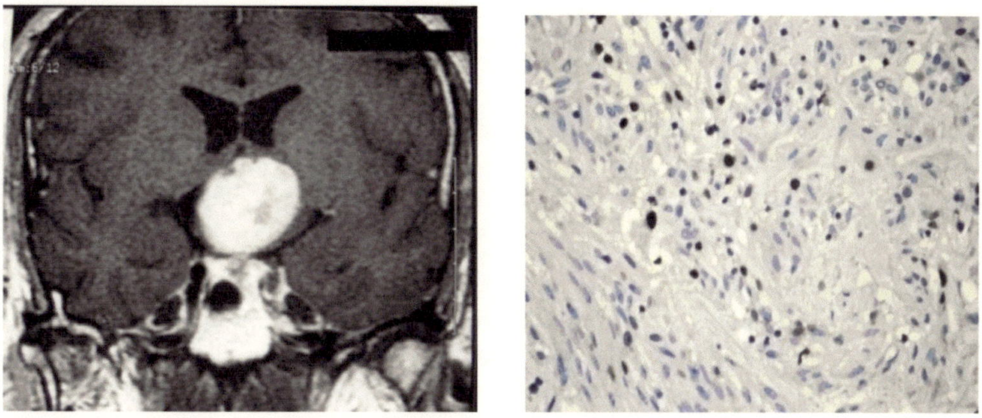

Figure 2. (Left) Representative appearance of chordoid glioma on MR imaging. Note a suprasellar mass occupying the anterior portion of the third ventricle and compressing the anterior ventricular floor on coronal contrast-enhanced T1-weighted and note high Ki-67 LI in neoplastic cells (right).

2.5. Challenges in diagnosing brain tumors

Obtaining brain tissue by the surgeon does not always guarantee that a final diagnosis will be reached, because unfortunately sampling errors or misinterpretation of the findings may still occur. Stereotaxic biopsy provides merely a trivial amount of material, and only the normal tissue or nonspecific anomalies such as gliosis or necrosis may be seen in the histological assessment. The use of spectroscopy, PET and SPECT for guiding biopsy reduces the sampling challenge [50]. However, it should not be forgotten that the biopsy comes from different clinics. Pathologists should also remember that there may be extraneuroaxial meningioma (**Figure 3**) in a patient with the symptom of a mass at the nasopharynx [51]. Paraffin block analysis unveils major histological characteristics; however, the findings may not meet all diagnostic criteria for the suspected disease. At this point, the pathologist may be obliged to make a choice between a report without an outcome and the outcome report comprising the most probable diagnosis although it does not meet all diagnostic criteria. Rather than having the clinician focus only on the outcome, ensuring that he/she reads the whole pathology report is important for the treatment to be aware of the unconfirmed grade of the histological diagnosis made [52].

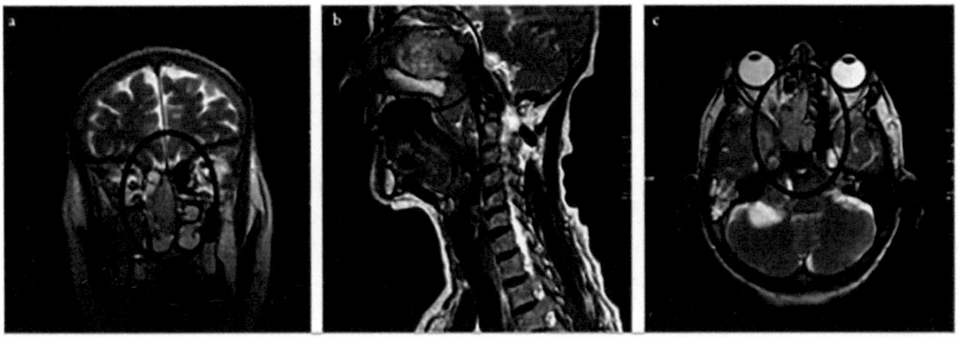

Figure 3. Coronal (a), sagittal (b) and axial (c) T2-sectional images of magnetic resonance imaging demonstrated a tumor beginning from the corner of the right cerebellopontine and extending along the nasopharynx-oropharynx-hypopharynx.

Accurate and timely diagnosis is the key principle in neuro-oncology [53]. Cancer treatment is often toxic; however, the risk of toxic effects is overlooked considering the potential gains in life expectancy when the appropriate treatment is administered to the right patient.

But, does the impact of each mass seen in the brain refer to a neoplasm? Diagnosing brain tumors is not crystal clear process. Many non-neoplastic neurological diseases may resemble brain neoplasms in the histological assessment or neuroimaging [54, 55]. In their review, Omura et al. [52] elaborated on differential diagnosis in these tumor-like lesions comprising multiple sclerosis, stroke, pyogenic abscess, toxoplasmosis, tuberculosis, cysticercosis, fungal infections, syphilis, sarcoidosis, Behçet's disease, radiation necrosis and venous thrombosis. They have detailed the elements supporting non-neoplastic diagnosis and helpful tips for differential diagnosis in brain lesions which uptake the contrast material. The findings which may support non-neoplastic diagnosis are as follows: sudden onset in young adults (AIDS), traveling to endemic countries (cysticercosis, hydatidosis), sexual behavior and use of drugs in IV form (AIDS, syphilis), history of autoimmune or inflammatory disease (MS, Behçet's disease, sarcoidosis), chronic fever, dental procedures (brain abscesses) transient neurologic deficits and vision symptoms (MS), and skin rashes (Behçet's disease, sarcoidosis, AIDS).

The vital questions in guiding the treatment, to be raised by pathologists at each biopsy, gained a critical importance once again with what has been described here. Is biopsy sufficient for diagnosis? If the material in sufficient, is it neoplastic or non-neoplastic? If the histological findings comply with the tumor, is this tumor primary or metastatic?

2.6. Detection and importance of metastatic brain tumors

Many pathologists/neuropathologists must have experienced a case similar to the one described below during intraoperative diagnosis. The tissue sampled from the mass in the brain during the operation by the surgeon is sent to the pathology lab for a frozen procedure. The pathologist who realizes the atypical pigmented cells tells the clinician doctor to seek for a lesion in the pigment of the patient's skin and tells that the microscopic finding matches melanoma; the surgeon reviews his/her patient and reports that, yes, there is an irregular skin lesion at a diameter of 2 cm in the lumbar region. Certainly, the diagnosis of metastatic lesions cannot be made at the blink of an eye as described here.

Metastases constitute the most important cause of death from cancer, including the CNS tumors. Metastasis in the central nervous system (CNS) forms a major part of the routine in neuropathology. The annual prevalence in the United States is 170,000, which corresponds to 10 times more the prevalence of primary malignant brain tumors. It is known that a central nervous system metastasis occurs during this process in 20–40% of the patients with systemic cancer [13, 14, 54–56].

Metastatic lesions mostly carcinomas constitute 1/4–1/2 of intracranial tumors. The most frequent primary organs are the lungs, breasts, skin (melanoma), kidneys and the gastrointestinal canal tumors, and these account for 80% of metastatic tumors [56, 57].

Metastases form sharply circumscribed masses localized usually in the gray-white matter junction area inside the brain and are frequently surrounded by an edema belt. The border between the brain parenchyma and the tumor is markedly circumscribed microscopically by the reactive gliosis surrounding the tumor.

In addition to the direct and local effects of metastases, also paraneoplastic syndromes may affect the peripheral and central nervous system and may sometimes emerge as findings which enable malignant tumors to be noticed clinically [58]. There are antibodies developed against tumor antigens in most patients with paraneoplastic syndrome. Some of patterns seen more frequently are provided below:

- *subacute cerebellar degeneration* causing ataxia and involving destruction, gliosis and mild inflammatory infiltration in Purkinje cells
- *limbic encephalitis* causing subacute dementia, concentrated in the medial temporal lobe, involving perivascular inflammatory infiltration, microglial nodules and some neuronal loss

- *subacute sensorial neuropathy* causing change in the sensation of pain as a result of inflammation along with the loss in sensorial neurons in the dorsal stem ganglions
- *sudden onset psychosis, catatonia, epilepsy and coma syndrome* associated with the antibodies developing against ovarian teratoma and *N*-methyl-D aspartate (NMDA) receptor [14, 15].

CNS metastases typically emerge during the late phase of systemic malignancies [59]. In a large-series retrospective study of metastatic brain tumors, the average interval between the primary tumor and metastatic brain tumor was 8.5 months and this displayed a significant variation from 4 months in lung cancers up to 37 months in melanoma [60].

Systemic treatment models are not very effective in treating metastatic tumors in the brain. This is due to the fact that the blood-brain barrier prevents most chemotherapeutic agents from passing to the brain parenchyma. While surgical methods and the administration of excision or radiotherapy may be partially effective in solitary brain metastases, the disease may become fatal in multiple metastatic lesions and/or typically small cell carcinoma and melanoma, and even when there is leptomeningeal involvement associated with breast cancer [61, 62].

Most brain metastases occur with hematogenous diffusion. As most of the CNS blood flow occurs toward the cerebrum, 80% of metastatic tumors are seen in this region. Cerebrum is followed by the cerebellum with 15%, brain stem with 5% and deep structures. The lesions mostly emerge in the gray matter, and especially, the gray-white matter composition is impacted. A higher amount of involvement is seen in the areas fed by the mid-cerebral artery [63, 64]. The parietal lobe is the most affected lobe where arterial border zones and especially mid, anterior and posterior cerebral arteries display continuity. Frontal and occipital lobes are other regions where metastatic lesions are seen. The masses localized in the brain stem, corpus callosum and the deep white matter have a low chance of being metastatic [65]. Retrograde spread is possible in rare cases via cranial nerves, especially in the neoplasms of head-neck squamous carcinoma and malignant salivary gland [66, 67].

Radiologically, the metastases from the sharply circumscribed masses in the brain parenchyma are often surrounded by a belt of edema. Sometimes, necrotic areas with dark color at the center, as in glioblastomas (GBMs), require differentiation from high-grade gliomas, lymphomas, abscesses and even large demyelinating plaques [68].

2.7. Differential diagnosis of metastases from primary CNS tumors

Pekmezci and Perry [69] presented the following detailed and significantly helpful information for pathologists in their comprehensive study published recently, entitled the Neuropathology of Metastasis: Excluding a Primary CNS Tumor as a First Step in the Diagnosis of Metastatic Brain Lesion. The information on malignancies, mostly hidden from pathologists by clinicians, is extremely beneficial especially in tissue diagnosis. However, even in patients with known cancer, 11% of these patients present with a solitary brain lesion and most of these are high-grade gliomas [70]. The microscopic characteristics of metastatic tumors usually resemble the primary tumor when the metastatic tumor is well differentiated and do not create problems in the diagnosis. However, poorly differentiated neoplasms in the brain parenchyma always require that high-grade gliomas undergo differential diagnosis, as with glioblastomas, especially when they are solitary.

Epithelioid or rhabdoid glioblastomas may resemble metastatic tumors or melanomas. Negative staining specific to melanoma and carcinoma and additional glial markers such as GFAP, OLIG2 and SOX2 solve this dilemma almost in all cases [71].

As most metastatic lesions appear with fibrous stroma histologically, their borders with the surrounding brain parenchyma are marked. Generally, they may be easily differentiated from primary brain tumors. Differential diagnosis problems occur occasionally with diffuse infiltrative glioma, choroid plexus tumors and medulloblastoma and hemangioblastoma in the cerebellum. Small cell, epithelioid and adenoid type glioblastoma may sometimes be confused with undifferentiated carcinoma. Furthermore, the degenerative changes which may be seen in the metastatic tumor may mimic glioblastoma. It is necessary to differentiate papillary adenocarcinoma metastasis from choroid plexus carcinoma. In this case, it should not be forgotten that choroid plexus carcinoma occurs in the young age group. Although rare cases are reported in adults, newly defined choroid plexus markers such as Kin 7.1 and stanniocalcin-1 may provide additional help [72]. As diffuse immunohistochemicals, the EMA antibody, diffuse, strong staining pattern and Ber EP4 positivity indicate metastases. Considering the benign behavior of hemangioblastoma, the differential diagnosis of cerebellar hemangioblastoma and metastatic renal carcinoma is important. Moreover, both tumors may be seen in the von Hippel-Lindau disease. The use of inhibin alfa, aquaporin1 and epithelial markers may differentiate these two tumors [73–75]. It has been reported in recent studies that the antibody aquaporin1 is a very reliable marker for hemangioblastoma and that its use with the antibody AE1/AE3 (for RCC) is useful in differentiating the two tumors. The differentiation of small cell carcinoma of the lung and medulloblastoma may be challenging in the cerebellum. Although it is reported that some medulloblastomas may display positivity in EMA and cytokeratin, EMA and cytokeratin are still the most reliable markers in differential diagnosis [76, 77].

The number of metastatic foci varies between cases. In the retrospective surgical review, 45.6% of the patients had solitary brain metastasis (one CNS lesion, without other systemic metastases), 26.5% had single brain metastasis (one CNS lesion with other systemic metastases), while the rest had two or more brain metastases [77].

When they see an intracranial tumor, pathologists should not report the tumor as a metastatic tumor or metastatic carcinoma without the need for providing details after deciding whether it is primary brain tumor or not. Reporting the origin and typing of the primary tumor in brain biopsy are important due to the following reasons. First of all, the period spent by the clinician for investigating the localization of the primary tumor will lead to a loss of time and be costly for the patient. Secondly, unnecessary surgery will be avoided in cancers such as metastatic germ cell tumor and lymphoma in which medical treatment will be administered. Again, due to the same reason, it will be beneficial to diagnose breast, prostate, ovarian and small cell lung carcinomas where chemotherapy is effective, based on the metastatic tumor. Finally, in patients with metastatic brain tumor, the long-term prognosis is based on various factors such as the tumor type, the dimension and number of metastatic foci, degree of diffusion of the primary tumor, the presence or absence of a metastatic tumor also in the other organs, the level of cognitive functions and the age of the patient. Thus, knowing the tumor type for the oncologist is critical in planning the treatment process [78]. It is aimed to make a diagnosis especially for metastatic tumors with unknown primary tumor with the introduction of immunohistochemical methods and a large variety of markers for routine use. Actually, considering the medical tests and procedures to be performed on the patient with a tumor in which the primary origin is unknown, the cost of immunohistochemical methods will be less. However, the most important topic to be discussed regarding this matter is the selection of suitable markers within this wide choice of antibodies and makes the most accurate diagnosis.

2.8. Immunohistochemical markers used in investigating the origin of brain tumors with unknown primary

Often, it is possible to make a morphological distinction alone between carcinoma, lymphoma and melanoma. However, when morphology is no sufficient, additional supportive methods are applied. Usually, starting with the general markers such as cytokeratin (carcinoma), S100 (melanoma, glioma) and leukocyte common antigen (lymphoma) is the first widely accepted step [79, 80]. If there is no staining with any of these symptoms, then it may sarcoma, germ cell tumors or primary CNS tumor [81].

***Elevation of cytokeratin expression*:** The most frequently used cytokeratin in pathology practice is AE1/AE3. AE1 enters into reaction with CK10, CK15, CK16 and CK19, while AE3 enters into reaction with CK1, CK6 and CK8 [82]. Both display staining almost in all carcinomas. However, AE1 enters into reaction also with normal, reactive and neoplastic astrocytes at the same time. Therefore, it will be useful to start with the cocktail antibody CAM5.2 which comprises CK8 and CK18 that are known as small molecular weight keratins. Cytokeratin 7 and 20 antibodies are other antibodies which are beneficial in the investigation of the origin [77, 79–83] (**Table 4**).

***Melanocytic markers*:** Malignant melanoma is among the tumors most frequently metastasizing to the brain. In some cases, the presence of malignant melanoma may first be detected when there is a brain metastasis. Metastatic malignant melanoma displays positive staining with S100 protein. However, as the S100 protein may be expressed also in neurons, reactive astrocytes, glioma, neurophils and the Schwann cells, the use of these tumors in brain metastases is rather limited. As a nuclear transcription factor, SOX10 is expressed in the neural crest, melanocytes and the glial and Schwann cells. While there is limited expression in the CNS, it has a considerably high sensitivity also to melanoma [84]. Moreover, the use of the antibodies Melan-A, HMB-45, tyrosinase and MITF is also recommended [85, 86].

***Glial fibrillary acidic protein (GFAP)*:** This antibody used very frequently in the neuropathology routine, normal, reactive and neoplastic astrocytes, normal ependymal cells, neoplastic ependymal cell processes and retinal Muller glial cells. Furthermore, it should not be forgotten that the Schwann cells, Kupffer cells, chondrocytes and myoepithelial cells may be GFAP positive [25, 87].

Rate of metastasis		CAM 5.2	CK7	CK20	TTF-1 (nuclear)	CK5/CK6	CD56	Melan-A, HMB-45, S100	GCDFP-15	CA125	CDX2 (nuclear)	Vimentin	CD10, RCCMa (nuclear)	Number of metastasis
50%	Lung non-small cell carcinoma	+	+	–	+	–	–	–	–	–	–	–	–	Multiple
	Lung small cell carcinoma	+/–	–	–	+	–	+	–	–	–	–	–	–	
	Squamous cell carcinoma	+	–	–	–	+	–	–	–	–	–	–	–	
11%	Melanoma	–	–	–	–	–	–	+	–	–	–	+	–	Multiple
15%	Breast carcinoma	+	+	–	–	–	–	–	+	–	–	–	–	Single
	Endometrial carcinoma	+	+	–	–	–	–	–	–	+	–	–	–	
10%	Renal cell carcinoma	+/–	–	–	–	–	–	–	–	–	–	+	+	Single
4%	Colorectal carcinoma	+	–	+	–	–	–	–	–	–	+	–	–	Single
	Gastric/gastroesophageal carcinoma	+	+/–	+/–	–	–	–	–	–	–	+/–	–	–	

+, positive; –, negative; +/–, can be positive or negative.

Table 4. Immunohistochemical signatures of common CNS metastatic neoplasms (adapted from Ref. [80]).

Organ-specific markers: The use of two well-known organ-specific markers, namely thyroglobulin and prostate-specific antigen (PSA) antibodies, is rather limited as the metastasis of thyroid and prostate cancer to the brain is very rare—thyroid transcription factor (TTF-1) is expressed by normal thyroid and lung epithelium. Therefore, other than squamous cell carcinoma, it is positive in most of adenocarcinoma, small cell carcinoma, poorly differentiated non-small cell carcinoma, neuroendocrine carcinoma and lung origin carcinoma [88]. However, TTF-1 expression was reported in a rare 3rd ventricle ependymoma [89]. Furthermore, its use with epithelial markers such as CK7 will be diagnostic, especially in the diagnosis of adenocarcinoma metastasis [25, 77, 79–83, 90]. CDX2 is a caudal-type gene encoding intestine-specific transcription factor expressed in the intestinal epithelium. Its use with cytokeratin 7 and 20 is beneficial in terms of differential diagnosis gastric, gastroesophageal, colorectal and mucinous ovarian adenocarcinoma metastases [25, 83, 91]. As an intermediate-sized basic cytokeratin, CK7 is positive in lung adenocarcinoma, breast, ovarian, pancreatic, biliary tract, endometrium, prostatic, thyroid, salivary gland and urinary bladder cancers. While the specificity of the gross cystic disease fluid protein 15 (GCDFP-15)—used for the differential diagnosis of metastatic breast carcinoma—is 99%, its sensitivity level is rather low (50%). A strong HER2 amplification (immunohistochemical or FISH) may provide support at diagnosis [92, 93].

3. Concluding remarks

- If a poorly differentiated intracranial tumor is detected, the age, localization, and clinical and neurological findings should be questioned at first stage.
- Consequently, differential diagnosis should be made with these findings, and hematoxylin and eosin sections (primary tumor, metastatic carcinoma/melanoma/lymphoma/sarcoma) and immunohistochemical analysis should be performed.
- In order to make an immunohistochemical differential diagnosis for carcinoma, it is recommended to investigate the cytokeratin 7/20 profile and organ-specific markers upon ensuring that it is carcinoma by selecting a more specific marker such as CAM5.2 at first stage.

In conclusion, pathologists are aware of their responsibility in neurosciences which is increasing in importance, know the value of a multidisciplinary approach in the management of brain tumors together with oncologists, surgeons and radiologists and play an important role in the administration of individualized molecular treatment in metastatic cancers such as lung, breast and melanoma cancer by using skillfully immunohistochemical arguments not only in the accurate diagnosis of primary tumors but even in tumors where the primary source cannot be identified radiologically.

http://dx.doi.org/10.5772/65911

Acknowledgements

I would like to thank Professor Aydın Sav for base of my neuropathology education, Professor Tarık Tihan and Professor Büge Öz for their supports.

Author details

Serdar Altınay

Address all correspondence to: drserdara@yahoo.com

Ministry of Health, University of Health Science, Bakırköy Dr. Sadi Konuk Training and Research Hospital, Department of Pathology, Istanbul, Turkey

References

[1] Bailey P, Cushing H: A classification of the tumors of the glioma group on a histogenetic basis with a correlated study of prognosis. Lippincott, Philadelphia, 1926.

[2] Zülch KJ (ed). Histological typing of tumours of the central nervous system. World Health Organization, Geneva, 1979.

[3] Kleihues P, Burger PC, Scheithauer BW: The new WHO classification of brain tumours. Brain Pathol. 1993;3:255–68. Review.

[4] Louis DN, Ohgaki H, Wiestler OD, Cavenee WK, et al.: The 2007 WHO classification of tumours of the central nervous system. Acta Neuropathol. 2007;114:97–109.

[5] Louis DN. The next step in brain tumor classification: "Let us now praise famous men"... or molecules? Acta Neuropathol. 2012;124:761–62. doi:10.1007/s00401-012-1067-4

[6] Cancer Genome Atlas Research Network: Compheresensive genomic characterization defines human glioblastoma genes and core pathways. Nature. 2008;455:1061.

[7] Mawrin C, Perry A: Pathological classification and molecular genetics of meningiomas. J Neurooncol. 2010;99:379–91. doi:10.1007/s11060-010-0342-2. Epub 2010 Sep 1. Review.

[8] Riemenschneider MJ, Jeuken JW, Wesseling P, Reifenberger G: Molecular diagnostics of gliomas: state of the art. Acta Neuropathol. 2010;120:567–84. doi:10.1007/s00401-010-0736-4. Epub 2010 Aug 17.

[9] Dubuc AM, Northcott PA, Mack S, Witt H, et al.: The genetics of pediatric brain tumors. Curr Neurol Neurosci Rep. 2010;10:215–23. doi:10.1007/s11910-010-0103-9. Review.

[10] Cho YJ, Tsherniak A, Tamayo P, Santagata S, et al.: Integrative genomic analysis of medulloblastoma identifies a molecular subgroup that drives poor clinical outcome. J Clin Oncol. 2011;29:1424–30. doi:10.1200/JCO.2010.28.5148. Epub 2010 Nov 22.

[11] Maher ER, Neumann HP, Richard S: von Hippel-Lindau disease: a clinical and scientific review. Eur J Hum Genet. 2011;19:617–23. doi:10.1038/ejhg.2010.175. Epub 2011 Mar 9. Review.

[12] Louis DN, Perry A, Burger P, Ellison DW, et al.: International Society of Neuropathology-Haarlem consensus guidelines for nervous system tumor classification and grading. Brain Pathol. 2014;24:429–35. doi:10.1111/bpa.12171

[13] Louis DN, Perry A, Reifenberger G, von Deimling A, et al.: The 2016 World Health Organization classification of tumors of the central nervous system: a summary. Acta Neuropathol. 2016;131:803–20. doi:10.1007/s00401-016-1545-1. Epub 2016 May 9. Review.

[14] Kumar V, Abbas AK: Robbins basic pathology. In: CNS tumors. 10th edition. Philadelphia, 2012.

[15] Perry A, Brat DJ: Practical surgical neuropathology. A diagnostic approach. Churchill Livingstone/Elsevier, Philadelphia, 2010.

[16] Burger PC, Scheithauer BW, et al.: Surgical pathology of the nervous system and ıts coverings. 4th edition. Churchill Livingstone, Philadelphia, 2002.

[17] Ostrom QT, Gittleman H, de Blank PM, Finlay JL, et al.: American Brain Tumor Association adolescent and young adult primary brain and central nervous system tumors diagnosed in the United States in 2008–2012. Neuro-Oncology. 2015;18:i1–i50. doi:10.1093/neuonc/nov297

[18] Altinay S, Sav A, Yapıcıer Ö, Elmacı İ: Ependymal tumors: correlation of proliferative (MIB-1), tumor suppressor (p53) and anti-apoptotic (bcl-2) indices with histologic types and grading. Acıbadem Univ J Health Sci. 2012;3:232–41.

[19] Clark HB. Immunohistochemistry of nervous system antigens: diagnostic applications in surgical neuropathology. Semin Diagn Pathol. 1984;1:309–16.

[20] Kleihues P, Kiessling M, Janzer RC: Morphological markers in neuro-oncology. Curr Top Pathol. 1987;77:307–38.

[21] Jaiswal S: Role of immunohistochemistry in the diagnosis of central nervous system tumors. Neurol India. 2016;64:502–12. doi:10.4103/0028-3886.181547

[22] Ueki K, Nishikawa R, Nakazato Y, Hirose T, et al.: Correlation of histology and molecular genetic analysis of 1p, 19q,10q, TP53, EGFR, CDK4, and CDKN2A in 91 astrocytic and oligodendroglial tumors. Clin Cancer Res. 2002;8:196–201.

[23] Ueki K: Oligodendroglioma: impact of molecular biology on its definition, diagnosis and management. Neuropathology. 2005;25:247–53.

[24] Trembath D, Miller CR, Perry A: Gray zones in brain tumor classification: evolving concepts. Adv Anat Pathol. 2008;15:287–97.

[25] Dunbar E, Yachnis AT: Glioma diagnosis: Immunohistochemistry and beyond. Adv Anat Pathol. 2010;17:187–201.

[26] Tihan T, Viglione M, Rosenblum MK, et al.: Solitary fibrous tumors in the central nervous system. A clinicopathologic review of 18 cases and comparison to meningeal hemangiopericytoma. Arch Pathol Lab Med. 2003;127:432–9.

[27] Bouvier C, et al.: Solitary fibrous tumors and hemangiopericytomas of the meninges: overlapping pathological features and common prognostic factors suggest the same spectrum of tumors. Brain Pathol. 2011;15. doi:10.1111/j.1750-3639.2011.00552

[28] Cerilli LA, Wick MR: Immunohistology of soft tissue and osseous neoplasms. In: Dabbs DJ (ed.) Diagnostic ımmunohistochemistry. Churchill Livingstone, Philadelphia, 2006, pp. 65–120.

[29] Park SH, Chang KH, Song IC, Kim YJ, Kim SH, Han MH: Diff usion-weighted MRI in cystic or necrotic intracranial lesions. Neuroradiology. 2000;42:716–21.

[30] Cha S: Perfusion MR imaging: basic principles and clinical applications. Magn Reson Imaging Clin N Am. 2003;11:403–13.

[31] Lasch P, Naumann D: FTIR microspectroscopic imaging of human carcinoma in thin sections based on pattern recognition techniques. Cell Mol. Biol. 1998;44:189–202.

[32] Krafft C, Shapoval L, Sobottka SB, Geiger KD, et al.: Identification of primary tumors of brain metastases by SIMCA classification of IR spectroscopic images. Biochim Biophys Acta. 2006;1758:883–91. Epub 2006 May 19.

[33] Kouwenhoven MC, Gorlia T, Kros JM, Ibdaih A, et al.: Molecular analysis of anaplastic oligodendroglial tumors in a prospective randomized study: a report from EORTC study 26951. Neuro Oncol. 2009;11:737–46.

[34] Hartmann C, von Deimling A: Molecular pathology of oligodendroglial tumors. Recent Results Cancer Res. 2009;171:25–49.

[35] Ohgaki H, Kleihues P: Genetic alterations and signalling pathways in the evolution of gliomas. Cancer Sci. 2009;100:2235–41.

[36] Molnár P: Classification of primary brain tumors: molecular aspects. In: Miklos Garami (ed.) Management of CNS Tumors. ISBN: 978-953-307-646-1. InTech. 2011. Available from: http://www.intechopen.com/books/management-of-cns- tumors/classification-of-primary-brain-tumorsmolecular-aspects

[37] Parsons DW, et al.: An ıntegrated genomic analysis of human glioblastoma multiforme. Science. 2008;321:1807–12.

[38] Balss J, Meyer J, et al.: Analysis of the IDH1 codon 132 mutation in brain tumors. Acta Neuropathol. 2008;116:597–602.

[39] Yan H, et al.: IDH1 and IDH2 mutations in gliomas. NEJM. 2009;360:13–21.

[40] Zhao Sh, et al.: Glioma-derived mutations in IDH1 dominantly ınhibit IDH1 catalytic activity and ınduce HIF-1α. Science. 2009;324:261–65.

[41] Dietel M, Jöhrens K, Laffert MV, Hummel M, et al.: A 2015 update on predictive molecular pathology and its role in targeted cancer therapy: a review focussing on clinical relevance. Cancer Gene Ther. 2015;22:417–30. doi:10.1038/cgt.2015.39. Epub 2015 Sep 11. Review.

[42] Aldape K, Burger PC, Perry A: Clinicopathologic aspects of 1p/19q loss and the diagnosis of oligodendroglioma. Arch Pathol Lab Med. 2007;131:242–51.

[43] Basaran R, Uslu S, Gucluer B, Onoz M, et al.: Impact of 1p/19q codeletion on the diagnosis and prognosis of different grades of meningioma. Br J Neurosurg. 2016;30:571–6. doi:10.1080/02688697.2016.1181155. Epub 2016 May 13.

[44] Cairncross G, Wang M, Shaw E, Jenkins R, et al.: Phase III trial of chemoradiotherapy for anaplastic oligodendroglioma: long-term results of RTOG 9402. J Clin Oncol. 2013;31:337–43.

[45] van den Bent MJ, Brandes AA, Taphoorn MJ, Kros JM, et al.: Adjuvant procarbazine, lomustine, and vincristine chemotherapy in newly diagnosed anaplastic oligodendroglioma: long-term follow-up of EORTC brain tumor group study 26951. J Clin Oncol. 2013;31:344–50.

[46] Malmstrom A, Gronberg BH, Marosi C, Stupp R, et al.: Temozolomide versus standard 6-week radiotherapy versus hypofractionated radiotherapy in patients older than 60 years with glioblastoma: the Nordic randomised, phase 3 trial. Lancet Oncol. 2012;13:916–26.

[47] Wick W, Platten M, Meisner C, Felsberg J, et al.: Temozolomide chemotherapy alone versus radiotherapy alone for malignant astrocytoma in the elderly: the NOA-08 randomised, phase 3 trial. Lancet Oncol. 2012; 3:707–15.

[48] van den Bent MJ, Dubbink HJ, Marie Y, Brandes AA: IDH1 and IDH2 mutations are prognostic but not predictive for outcome in anaplastic oligodendroglial tumors: a report of the European Organization for Research and Treatment of Cancer Brain Tumor Group. Clin Cancer Res. 2010;16:1597–604.

[49] Altınay S, Sav A, Özduman K, Kılıç T.: Chordoid glioama of the third ventricle with high MIB-1 index. J Clin Exp Pathol. 2015;5. doi:10.4172/2161-0681.1000235

[50] Sawin PD, Hitchon PW, Follett KA, Torner JC: Computed imaging-assisted stereotactic brain biopsy. A risk analysis of 225 consecutive cases. Surg Neurol. 1998;49:640–9.

[51] Altınay S, Belli Ş, Şentürk T, Toksöz M, et al.: A case of cranial meningioma with symptoms similar to nasopharyngeal mass. Turk Arch Otorhinolaryngol. 2015;53:90–2. doi:10.5152/tao.2015.603

[52] Omuro AM, Leite CC, Mokhtari K, Delattre JY: Pitfalls in the diagnosis of brain tumours. Lancet Neurol. 2006;5:937–48. doi:10.1016/S1474-4422(06)70597-X

[53] Behin A, Hoang-Xuan K, Carpentier AF, Delattre JY: Primary brain tumours in adults. Lancet. 2003;361:323–31.

[54] Lassman AB, DeAngelis LM: Brain metastases. Neurol Clin. 2003;21:1–23.

[55] Okamoto K, Furusawa T, Ishikawa K, Quadery FA, et al.: Mimics of brain tumor on neuroimaging: part II. Radiat Med. 2004;22:135–42.

[56] Barnholtz-Sloan JS, Sloan AE, Davis FG, Vigneau FD, et al.: Incidence proportions of brain metastases in patients diagnosed (1973 to 2001) in the Metropolitan Detroit Cancer Surveillance System. J Clin Oncol. 2004;22:2865–72.

[57] Nayak L, Lee EQ, Wen PY: Epidemiology of brain metastases. Curr Oncol Rep. 2012;14:48–54.

[58] Giordana MT, Cordera S, Boghi A: Cerebral metastases as first symptom of cancer: a clinico-pathologic study. J Neurooncol. 2000;50:265–73.

[59] Zimm S, Wampler GL, Stablein D, Hazra T, et al.: Intracerebral metastases in solid-tumor patients: natural history and results of treatment. Cancer. 1981;48:384–94.

[60] Lagerwaard FJ, Levendag PC, Nowak PJ, Eijkenboom WM, et al.: Identification of prognostic factors in patients with brain metastases: a review of 1292 patients. Int J Radiat Oncol Biol Phys. 1999;43:795–803.

[61] Sheehan J, Niranjan A, Flickinger JC, et al.: The expanding role of neurosurgeons in the management of brain metastases. Surg Neurol. 2004;62:32–40.

[62] Chamberlain MC: Leptomeningeal metastasis. Curr Opin Neurol. 2009;22:665–74.

[63] Delattre JY, Krol G, Thaler HT, Posner JB: Distribution of brain metastases. Arch Neurol. 1988;45:741–4.

[64] Nathoo N, Chahlavi A, Barnett GH, et al.: Pathobiology of brain metastases. J Clin Pathol. 2005;58:237–42.

[65] Patchell RA: The management of brain metastases. Cancer Treat Rev. 2003;29:533–40.

[66] Nussbaum ES, Djalilian HR, Cho KH, Hall WA: Brain metastases. Histology, multiplicity, surgery, and survival. Cancer. 1996;78:1781–8.

[67] Spencer ML, Neto AG, Fuller GN, Luna MA: Intracranial extension of acinic cell carcinoma of the parotid gland. Arch Pathol Lab Med. 2005;129:780–2.

[68] Rong Y, Durden DL, Van Meir EG, Brat DJ: 'Pseudopalisading' necrosis in glioblastoma: a familiar morphologic feature that links vascular pathology, hypoxia and angiogenesis. J Neuropathol Exp Neurol. 2006;65:529–39.

[69] Pekmezci M, Perry A: Neuropathology of brain metastases. Surg Neurol Int. 2013;4:245–55. doi:10.4103/2152-7806.111302. Print 2013.

[70] Patchell RA, Tibbs PA, Walsh JW, Dempsey RJ, et al.: A randomized trial of surgery in the treatment of single metastases to the brain. N Engl J Med.1990;322:494–500.

[71] Oliver-De La Cruz J, Carrión-Navarro J, García-Romero N, Gutiérrez-Martín A, et al.: SOX2+ cell population from normal human brain white matter is able to generate mature oligodendrocytes. PLoS One. 2014;9:e99253. doi:10.1371/journal.pone.0099253. eCollection 2014.

[72] Hasselblatt M, Bohm C, Tatenhorst L, Dinh V, et al.: Identification of novel diagnostic markers for choroid plexus tumors: a microarray-based approach. Am J Surg Pathol. 2006;30:66–74.

[73] Carney EM, Banerjee P, Ellis CL, Albadine R, et al.: PAX2(−)/PAX8(−)/inhibin A(+) immunoprofile in hemangioblastoma: a helpful combination in the differential diagnosis with metastatic clear cell renal cell carcinoma to the central nervous system. Am J Surg Pathol. 2011;35:262–7.

[74] Mena H, Ribas JL, Pezeshkpour GH, et al.: Hemangiopericytoma of the central nervous system: a review of 94 cases. Hum Pathol. 1991;22:84–91.

[75] Weinbreck N, et al.: Immunohistochemical markers to distinguish between hemangioblastoma and metastatic clear-cell renal cell carcinoma in the brain: utility of aquaporin1 combined with cytokeratin AE1/AE3 ımmunostaining. Am J Surg Pathol. 2008;32:1051–59.

[76] Pinkus GS, Kurtin PJ: Epithelial membrane antigen. A diagnostic discriminant in surgical pathology. Immunohiostochemical profile in epithelial, mesenchymal, and hematopoietic neoplasms using paraffin sections and monoclonal antibodies. Hum Pathol. 1985;16:929–40.

[77] Chu PG, Weiss LM: Keratin expression in human tissues and neoplasms. Histopathology. 2002;40:403–39.

[78] Stark AM, Stohring C, Hedderich J, Held-Feindt J, et al.: Surgical treatment for brain metastases: prognostic factors and survival in 309 patients with regard to patient age. J Clin Neurosci. 2011;18:34–8.

[79] Dabbs DJ: Immunohistology of metastatic carcinoma of unknown primary. In: Dabbs DJ (ed) Diagnostic immunohistochemistry. Churchill Livingstone, Philadelphia, 2006, pp. 180–226.

[80] Becher MW, Abel TW, Thompson RC, Weaver KD, et al.: Immunohistochemical analysis of metastatic neoplasms of the central nervous system. J Neuropathol Exp Nerol. 2006;65:935–44. doi:10.1097/01.jnen.0000235124.82805.2b

[81] Drlicek M, Bodenteich A, Urbanits S, et al.: Immunohistochemical panel of antibodies in the diagnosis of brain metastases of the unknown primary. Pathol Res Pract. 2004;200:727–34.

[82] Moll R, Franke WW, Schiller DL, et al.: The catalog of human cytokeratins: patterns of expression in normal epithelia, tumors and cultured cells. Cell. 1982;31:11–24.

[83] Taweevisit M, Isarakul P, Chaipipat M, Keetacheeva K, et al.: Cytokeratin 7 and 20 as immunohistochemical markers in identification of primary tumors in craniospinal metastases: do they have a significant role? Neuropathology. 2003;23:271–4.

[84] Shin J, Vincent JG, Cuda JD, Xu H, et al.: Sox 10 is expressed in primary melanocytic neoplasms of various histologies but not in fibrohistiocytic proliferations and histiocytoses. J Am Acad Dermatol. 2012;67:717–26.

[85] Zimmer C, Gottschalk J, Goebel S, et al.: Melanoma-associated antigens in tumours of the nervous system: an immunohistochemical study with the monoclonal antibody HMB-45. Virchows Arch A Pathol Anat Histopathol. 1992;420:121–26.

[86] Takeda K, Yasumoto K, Takada R, et al.: Induction of melanocytespecific microphthalmia-associated transcription factor by Wnt-3a. J Biol Chem. 2000;275:14013–16.

[87] de Armond SJ, Eng LF, Rubinstein LJ: The application of glial fibrillary acidic (GFA) protein immunohistochemistry in neurooncology. A progress report. Pathol Res Pract. 1980;168:374–94.

[88] Srodon M, Westra WH: Immunohistochemical staining for thyroid transcription factor-1: a helpful aid in discerning primary site of tumor origin in patients with brain metastases. Hum Pathol. 2002;33:642–5.

[89] Zamecnik J, Chanova M, Kodet R: Expression of thyroid transcription factor 1 in primary brain tumours. J Clin Pathol. 2004;57:1111–3.

[90] Ramaekers F, van Niekerk C, Poels L, Schaafsma E, et al.: Use of monoclonal antibodies to keratin 7 in the differential diagnosis of adenocarcinomas. Am J Pathol. 1990;136:641–55.

[91] Werling RW, Yaziji H, Bacchi CE, Gown AM: CDX2, a highly sensitive and specific marker of adenocarcinomas of intestinal origin: an immunohistochemical survey of 476 primary and metastatic carcinomas. Am J Surg Pathol. 2003;27:303–10.

[92] Wick MR, Lillemoe TJ, Copland GT, Swanson PE, et al.: Gross cystic disease fluid protein-15 as a marker for breast cancer: ımmunohistochemical analysis of 690 human neoplasms and comparison with alpha-lactalbumin. Hum Pathol. 1989;20:281–7.

[93] Greco FA, Lennington WJ, Spigel DR, Hainsworth JD: Molecular profiling diagnosis in unknown primary cancer: accuracy and ability to complement standard pathology. J Natl Cancer Inst. 2013; 105: 782–790.

Section 3

Radiation Therapies for CNS Malignancies

Chapter 3

A Review of Current Radiation Therapies for the Treatment of Metastatic Brain Tumors

Jonathan S. Hayman

Additional information is available at the end of the chapter

http://dx.doi.org/10.5772/65869

Abstract

The treatment of brain tumors has evolved over the past few decades. While whole brain radiation therapy was the standard of care in the management of tumors for years, stereotactic radiation has for the most part replaced the technique in the management of metastatic tumors of the brain. In this review, the current indications are reviewed for both whole brain and stereotactic radiation therapy in the management of metastatic cancers involving the central nervous system, the most common types of malignancies diagnosed in the brain.

Keywords: radiosurgery, whole brain radiation, prophylactic cranial radiation, history of cranial radiation

1. Introduction

The incidence of metastatic cancer involving the CNS is increasing and was >220,000 cases in the US alone in 2015, >20 times the incidence of high grade glioblastoma (GBM) [1, 2]. The four most common tumor types that metastasized to the brain were *lung* > *breast* > *melanoma* > *renal cell*—1,2,3,4, with median survival worse than those reported for primary CNS malignancies—8 *vs*. 13 months for GBM [1–4].

This increase in CNS involvement may be associated with the increased survival associated with improved therapy for the primary sites, permitting micrometastases in the CNS to become apparent. The management of CNS metastases remains ineffective [1, 2]. Thus, 'subjects are living longer with cancer', but also, and perhaps as a consequence, have an increased risk of developing metastases involving the CNS—a 'safe haven' from systemic chemotherapy [4].

The incidence of intracranial metastases observed at the times of autopsy was reported half a century ago and revealed that 5% of subjects with all types of cancer possessed brain metastases [5]. In the 1950s, the diagnosis of cancer involving the brain was made from clinical symptoms such as headaches, confusion, seizures, etc. and confirmed by physical findings such as papilledema hemiplegia, ataxia and aphasia. Further evidence could be obtained by electroencephalograms (EEG) and later carotid angiography and nuclear brain scanning were used [5]. With the advent of 'computerized axial tomography' (CT) and 'magnetic resonance imaging' (MRI), more exact delineation of the degrees of brain involvement is now possible, and higher incidences of metastatic brain disease are now appreciated [2, 4].

2. Radiation therapy

Radiation therapy (RT) has been the mainstay in the management of CNS metastases. Since the presentation is often multi-focal, surgery is not indicated [4]. However, responses of tumor metastases to whole brain radiation therapy (WBRT) (the current standard of care) are usually incomplete and of short duration and often accompanied by local toxicities, such as neurocognitive loss, etc. [4].

Whole brain radiation therapy (WBRT) was the treatment of choice in the past [6]. WBRT was usually started with a warm up dose of 50 cGy on the first treatment day increasing gradually to 200 cGy over several daily fractions to a planned total dose of 3000–4000 cGy [6].

The advent of glucocorticoid steroids controlled the radiation side effects such as headaches, papilledema, etc. and allowed higher daily doses of radiation to be given without exacerbation of intracranial edema, etc. [7, 8]. Although palliative care was provided, neurocognitive and other neurological/behavioral disorders still existed [9]. Also, the doses of WBRT administered were insufficient to treat subclinical metastatic disease that is not seen on the imaging tools available. The common dose schedules used were 3000 cGy in 10 fractions or 4000 cGy in 16 fractions [6].

With improved knowledge regarding tumor biology and more comprehensive tumor registries, certain tumors were found to have a higher propensity for brain metastasis—*lung* > *breast* > *melanoma* > *renal cell*—1,2,3,4 [4]. In subjects with these types of tumors prone to brain metastases, prophylactic brain radiation at lower doses began to be included in subject care plans. The goals have always been to kill off microscopic involvement, improve disease free survival with improved quality of life (QOL) and diminish morbidities associated with brain metastases.

2.1. Radiosurgical devices

With the development of radiosurgical instruments such as the Gamma Knife and Cyber Knife, it is possible to radiate individual metastatic lesions with great accuracy. In combination with MRI techniques, stereotactic radiosurgery (SRS) has become the most widely used procedure to reduce metastatic CNS cancer lesions and has also reduced the incidence of radiation-associated neurocognitive effects [9–13]. The exact radiation dosing varies depending on the size and number of metastases [13, 14]. As these techniques have improved, combining

WBRT with SRS has been evaluated, and after multiple studies, no increase in overall survival (OS) (but an increase in local control) with WBRT after surgery/radiosurgery has been observed [15–18]. However, there still remains scenarios in which WBRT may be beneficial. Later in the chapter, we will review this evidence for the use of WBRT.

3. Adjuvant or prophylactic cranial irradiation (PCI)

3.1. History and rationale

The recognition that certain cancer cell types have a propensity to spread to the central nervous system created interest in adjuvant or prophylactic cranial irradiation (PCI) for some malignancies at lower therapeutic doses [7, 18, 19].

3.2. Childhood leukemia: PCI

In children with acute leukemia, it was recognized that the CNS is a sanctuary site for malignant cells and PCI became the standard therapy for many years [19–22]. However, because of the neurocognitive/behavioral defects and the decrease in IQs that were noted in children who received PCI for childhood leukemia, other treatment methodologies were compared with and without radiation [20]. In 2003, a meta-analysis of 43 randomized trials concluded that radiotherapy can be replaced by long-term intrathecal therapy and a 2009 prospective randomized trial confirmed with 501 subjects confirmed that radiation can be omitted from treatment [21, 22]. As such, PCI in the setting of leukemia is not routinely used in clinical practice.

3.3. Small cell lung cancer: PCI

Small cell carcinoma of the lung (SCLC) has a propensity to metastasize to the brain and CNS, where there has been great enthusiasm for the use of PCI. NCCN guidelines still support its use [7, 8, 23, 24]. However, due to the associated neurodegeneration, there is a trend to only treat the brain with radiation, if lesions are detected [23]. The original rationale for prophylactic cranial irradiation (PCI) in limited small cell cancer that was advocated by Hansen in 1973 is that CNS relapse in small cell lung cancer is analogous to isolated CNS relapse in Acute lymphoblastic leukemia (ALL) [7].

The first meta-analysis published by Prophylactic Cranial Irradiation Overview Collaborative Group supporting the use of PCI in limited SCLC was published in 1999 and proved that PCI reduced the incidence of brain metastases by 50% with an absolute survival advantage of 5%. This 5% was the same amount of absolute survival advantage seen with thoracic radiation after induction chemotherapy in limited SCLC [25].

Of importance, a high proportion of subjects with SCLC had specific cognitive defects prior to PCI without any significant deterioration following PCI. For extensive SCLC, the European Organization for Research and Treatment of Cancer (EORTC) Lung Cancer Group showed a slight improvement in survival with the addition of PCI after induction therapy, but in absolute terms, the benefit was minimal after 1 year; survival in the radiated group was 27.1%, as compared with 13.3% in the control group. In the PCI group, two subjects remained alive at 24 months, while in the control (no PCI), all subjects were dead by 18 months [24].

NCCN treatment guidelines continue to recommend PCI for SCLC, even though there have been significant advances in the imaging and treatment of brain metastases. Since many of the original studies advocating the use of PCI were published using CT as the imaging choice for the brain, it is now postulated that many small brain metastases that were missed by CT would have been detected by sensitive MRI [8]. The fact that MRI scanning detects SCLC metastasis 24% of the time, as opposed to 11% with CT, means that there will be fewer patients with undetected cranial metastases after imaging with a contrast-enhanced MRI study, thus possibly reducing the role for WBRT going forward.

There is also a greater awareness of the potential deleterious effects of whole brain irradiation on stem cell and immune modulating cell compartments within the brain, the importance of which in humans was originally reported in 1998 [25]. This observation encouraged the development of techniques to limit radiation dose to critical structures such as the hippocampus and sub-ventricular zone [26–28]. Currently, a Phase 3 trial—NRG-CC003: A Randomized Phase II/III Trial of Prophylactic Cranial Irradiation with or without Hippocampal Avoidance for Small Cell Lung Cancer—is comparing partial cranial radiation with and without sparing of the hippocampus in subjects with small cell lung cancer (SCLC) involving the brain, will be completed by 2019 [26].

As such, the guidelines for PCI in limited SCLC may change within the next few years. Since there is improvement in survival with PCI, the benefits and risks should be discussed with each subject to allow them to determine if they want the therapy.

3.4. Non-small cell lung cancer (NSCLC): PCI

NSCLC is the most common cancer to metastasize to the brain and 7.4% of subjects with NSCLC have brain metastases at presentation of primary disease [4]. Another 25–30% of the subjects with NSCLC will develop brain metastases during the course of their disease [2, 27]. Because of the improvement in absolute survival seen in limited SCLC, the radiation therapy oncology group (RTOG) has performed two trials of prophylactic cranial radiation in NSCLC cancer.

The first RTOG trial study population included 161 subjects treated for medically or surgically inoperable primary cancers and 26 subjects undergoing adjuvant postoperative mediastinal irradiation following attempted curative resection of primary cancers found to have metastasized to hilar or mediastinal lymph nodes [28]. Published in 1991, the 94 subjects randomized to chest irradiation alone had a 19% incidence of brain metastases. In subjects randomized to receive prophylactic cranial irradiation, there was a 9% incidence of brain metastases. Despite the dramatic improvement in local control of brain disease, no survival difference was observed between the treatment arms. Because of the absence of reliable therapy for the primary disease at that time and the lack of effective systemic therapy to prevent dissemination to extra-thoracic sites, prophylactic cranial irradiation for inoperable NSCLC was not justified in routine clinical practice [28].

A more recent RTOG study evaluating PCI in NSCLC was published in 2011 [29]. RTOG 0214 was performed with subjects that had locally advanced NSCLC. Subject eligibility was Stage III NSCLC without disease progression after treatment with surgery and/or radiation therapy

(RT) with or without chemotherapy. This study showed a decrease in brain metastases in the PCI group [7.7% (PCI cohort) at 1 year *vs.* 18.0% (observation) at 1 year]. However, there was no effects on survival due to the devastating effects of systemic NSCLC without effective systemic therapy The disease free survival and overall survival were essentially the same (1 year OS 75.6 *vs.* 76.9%; DFS 56.4 *vs.* 51.2%) [29].

In another study, Sun *et al.* reviewed the neuropsychiatric profiles for these subjects and showed that, although PCI did not significantly impact overall reported quality of life PCI in Stage III NSCLC, did not reduce global cognitive function or quality of life (QOL), and there was a significant decline in memory at 1 year in the PCI group [30]. Given that there is no survival benefit from PCI in NSCLC and that there is cognitive toxicity, at the present time, PCI is not recommended by the NCCN for NSCLC [31].

4. Metastatic brain carcinoma

Historically, the treatment of metastatic brain disease was whole brain radiation ranging in doses of 2000 cGy in 5 fractions to 4000 cGy in 16 fractions [3]. This resulted in good palliation and reduction of steroid dosage, but poor local control. Studies have shown an improvement in symptoms in 64–83% of subjects after treatment with WBRT alone and have also demonstrated an increase in median overall survival (OS) from 1 month with no treatment to 3–7 months following WBRT [32]. When reviewing data contained within studies of metastatic brain disease in the RTOG, control of disease is accomplished in approximately 50% of subjects at 6 months [32].

The development of radiosurgical techniques for brain lesions paralleled the studies of metastatic cancer involving brain conducted by the RTOG [32]. In 1987, the first report study of 12 patients who were treated with radiosurgery using a linear accelerator for brain metastases with a dose of at least 2000 cGy was presented [33].

With the advent of CT and MRI neuroradiologic imaging, the computer revolution allowed better planning of treatments and radiosurgery began to be used in earnest for treatment of brain metastases because of the knowledge that whole brain radiation had a failure rate of about 60% [2–4].

Many studies have been reported for SRS and RTOG recursive partitioning analysis (RPA) that was derived from studies of whole brain radiation and the use of radiation sensitizers [33]. This platform analysis has allowed a better appreciation of results [33].

Recursive partitioning analysis (RPA) and statistical analysis has created a regression tree according to prognostic significance. Eighteen pretreatment characteristics and three treatment-related variables were analyzed. The RPA tree is based on four parameters (age, Karnofsky performance status (KPS), presence or absence of extracranial metastases and the control status of the primary tumor). The best survival (median: 7.1 months) was observed in subjects < 65 years of age with a Karnofsky Performance Status (KPS) of at least 70 and a controlled primary tumor with the brain the only site of metastases. The worst survival (median: 2.3 months) was seen in subjects with a KPS < 70. The following three classes are delineated: Class 1: subjects with KPS ≥ 70, <65 years of age with controlled primary and no extra cranial metastases; Class 2: KPS < 70; Class 3: all other subjects who were not 1 or 3. Using these classes or stages, new treatment techniques can be tested on homogeneous subject groups.

The important point regarding RPA is that if subjects are randomized in the same RPA class group two treatments can be compared without worry that differences in survival were due to subject selection. Numerous studies have been published in the field of radiosurgery for brain metastases, and it is beyond the scope of this chapter to provide a detailed analysis.

A decision platform from 'Intracranial Stereotactic Radiosurgery' shows appropriate management for patients with 1 and 2–4 brain metastasis in 2016 (**Figure 1**) [32, 33].

Chart 1

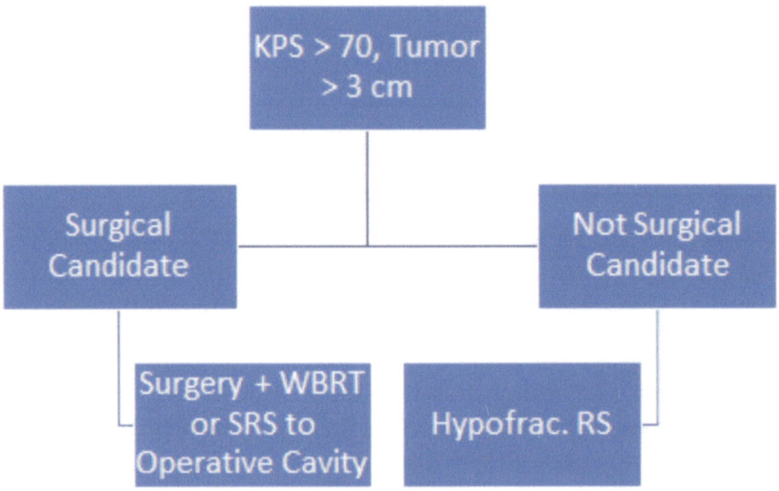

Chart 2

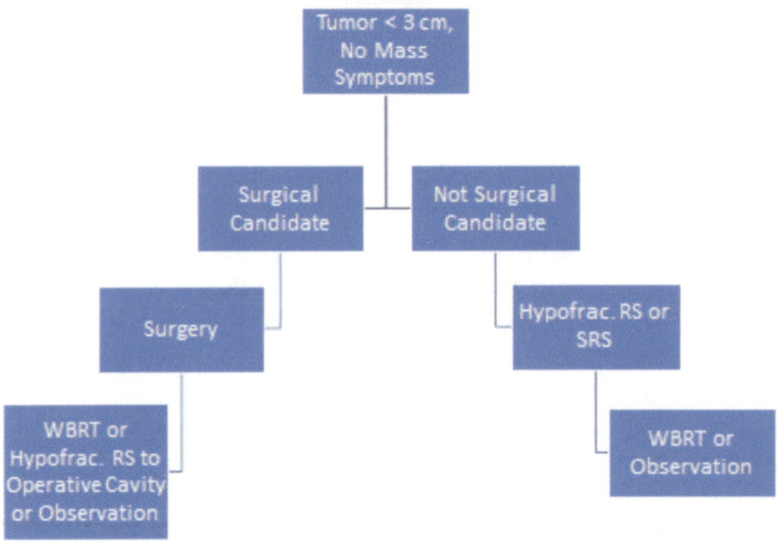

http://dx.doi.org/10.5772/65869

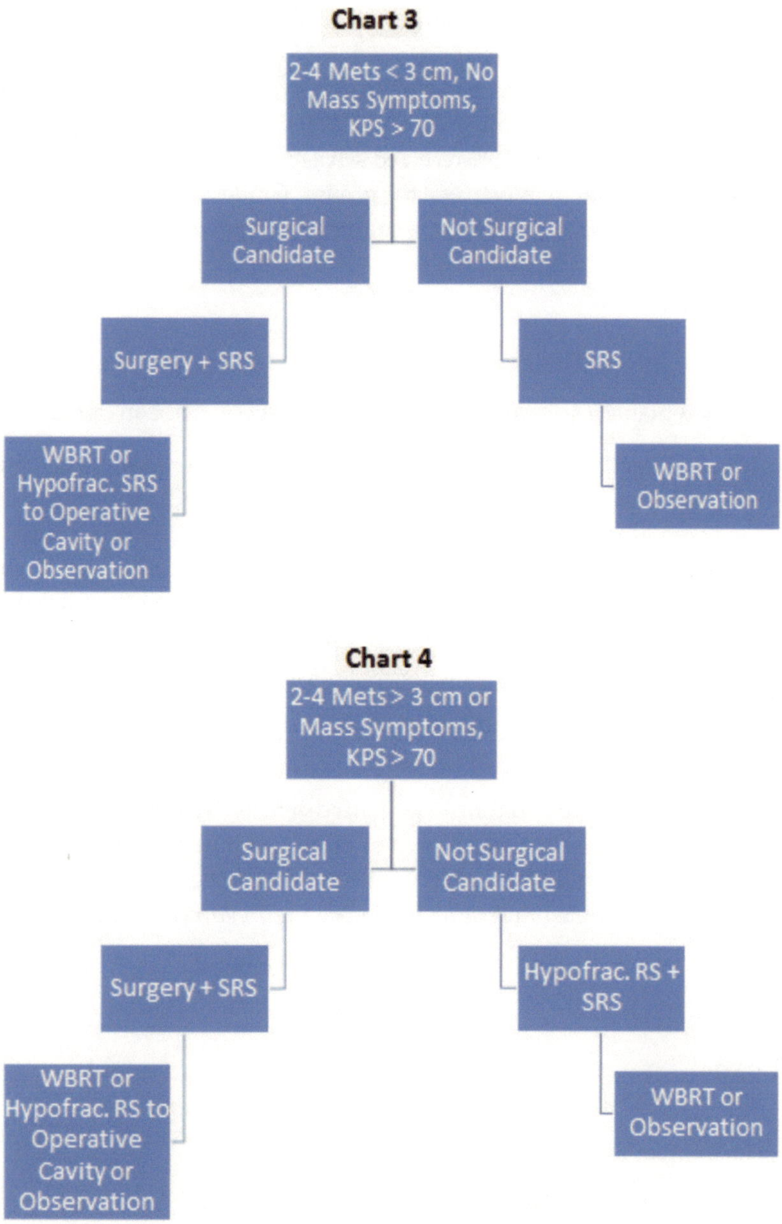

Figure 1. Flow chart for treatment of metastatic brain lesions.

Patients that have ≥5 metastatic lesions involving the brain have not been studied in any randomized trials. This is unfortunate because survival has varied considerably due to subject selection [33]. There is one randomized study group in Japan, which was a multi-institutional prospective study that included 1194 patients (76% with lung cancer). The aim was to examine whether survival after SRS without WBRT as initial treatment for subjects with 5–10 brain metastases (median 6) was inferior to that of patients with 2–4 lesions. Size limits were metastases <3 cm in longest diameter, largest tumor <10 ml in volume and total cumulative volume ≤15 ml. Median survival was longest in subjects with one lesion ($n = 455$, 13.9 months). However, subjects with 2–4 lesions had comparable survival to subjects with 5–10 lesions (median survival 10.8 months, hazard ratio 0.97, 95% confidence interval 0.81–1.18). This met the pre-specified definition of non-inferiority, despite the development of new lesions in >60% of subjects. Further salvage SRS was done in more than 40%, and 9% received salvage WBRT. The delivery of further SRS or WBRT was not significant different between the groups. Grade 3–4 adverse events occurred in up to 3% of subjects in each group; only 8% of subjects died from their brain disease [34].

5. Conclusion

Radiation therapy remains a secondary therapy when surgery is not an option.

Several facts have emerged. Local control of brain metastases does not translate into increased survival, although there may be long-term survivors in the RTOG RPA Class 1. Stereotactic radiosurgery with or without whole brain radiation is appropriate in the treatment of patients with 1–3 metastasis. Whole brain radiation when combined with SRS may have long-term deleterious effects on neuro-cognition. In combination with the newer immunomodulators, WBRT and/or SRS therapy may improve the usefulness of radiation [35].

The main three questions that remain to be answered regarding the treatment of metastatic brain disease focus on avoidance of toxicity from brain radiation through tissue sparing and dose reduction.

Can hippocampal sparing help avoid neurocognitive deficits? Will the development of novel radiosensitizers allow the use of lower doses of radiation and still achieve strong immune modulation? Can more sensitive MRI better define the extent of cancer metastases in the CNS and obviate the need for whole brain radiation in SCLC and ALL subjects.

All good questions to be answered in future randomized clinical trials with WBRT *vs*. SRS.

Author details

Jonathan S. Hayman

Address all correspondence to: haymanjs@gmail.com

Johns Hopkins Bayview Medical Center, Baltimore, MD, USA

References

[1] Chaubet-Houdu M, *Baseball*, Pechoux, C, Le Chevalier T. Management of brain metastases in non-small cell lung cancer. Cancer Chemother Rev, 7–15, 2012.

[2] Lin J, Jandial R, Nesbit A, Badie B, Chen M. Current and emerging treatments forbrain metastases. Oncology, 52: 250–268, 2015.

[3] Shankar G, Cahill DP. Management of brain metastases. ASCO Post, Jan15, 40–48, 2013.

[4] Termini J, Neman J, Jandial R. Role of the neural niche in brain metastatic cancer. Cancer Res, 74: 4011–4015, 2014.

[5] Willis R. The Spread of Tumours in the Human Body [2nd ed]. London. Butterworth & Co., Ltd. 1952; p. 255.

[6] Chao J-H, Phillips R, Nickson, JJ. Roentgen-ray therapy of cerebral metastases. Cancer, 7: 682–689, 1954.

[7] Hansen H. Should initial treatment of small cell carcinoma include systemic chemotherapy and brain irradiation? Cancer Chem Rep, 4: 239–241,1973.

[8] Seute T, et al. Detection of brain metastases from small cell lung cancer. Cancer, 112: 1827–1834, 2008.

[9] Crossen JR, *et al.* Neurobehavioral sequelae of cranial irradiation in adults: a review of radiation-induced encephalopathy. J Clin Oncol, 12: 627–642, 1994.

[10] Giovagnoli AR, Boiardi A. Cognitive impairment and quality of life in long-term survivors of malignant brain tumors. Ital J Neurol Sci, 15: 481–488, 1954.

[11] Johannesen TB, *et al.* Radiological and clinical assessment of long-term brain tumour survivors after radiotherapy. Radiother Oncol, 692: 169–176, 1954.

[12] Meyers CA, Brown PD. Role and relevance of neurocognitive assessment in clinical trials of patients with CNS tumors. J Clin Oncol, 24: 1305–1309, 2006.

[13] Jawahar A, *et al.* Gamma knife surgery in the management of brain metastases from lung carcinoma: a retrospective analysis of survival, local tumor control, and freedom from new brain metastasis. J Neurosurg, 100: 842–847, 2004.

[14] Adler JR, *et al.* Stereotactic radiosurgical treatment of brain metastases. J Neurosurg, 76: 444–449, 1992.

[15] Kocher M, *et al.* Adjuvant whole-brain radiotherapy versus observation after radiosurgery or surgical resection of one to three cerebral metastases: results of the EORTC 22952-26001 study. J Clin Oncol, 29: 134–141, 2011.

[16] Skibber JM, Soong SJ, Austin L, Balch CM, Sawaya RE. Cranial irradiation after surgical excision of brain metastases in melanoma patients. Ann Surg Oncol, 3: 118–123, 1996.

[17] Hagen NA, Cirrincione C, Thaler HT, DeAngelis LM. The role of radiation therapy following resection of single brain metastasis from melanoma. Neurology, 40: 158–160, 1990.

[18] Armstrong JG, Wronski M, Galicich J, Arbit E, Leibel SA, Burt M. Postoperative radiation for lung cancer metastatic to the brain. J Clin Oncol, 12: 2340–2344, 1994.

[19] Dahl GV, *et al.* Preventive central nervous system irradiation in children with acute nonlymphocytic leukemia. Cancer, 42: 2187–2219, 1978.

[20] Conklin HM, *et al.* Cognitive outcomes following contemporary treatment without cranial irradiation for childhood acute lymphoblastic leukemia. J Natl Canc Inst, 104: 1386–1395, 2012.

[21] Clarke M, *et al.* CNS-directed therapy for childhood acute lymphoblastic leukemia: childhood ALL collaborative group overview of 43 randomized trials. J Clin Oncol, 21: 1798–1809, 2003.

[22] Pui C-H, *et al.* Treating childhood acute lymphoblastic leukemia without cranial irradiation. N Engl J Med, 360: 2730–2741, 2009.

[23] Skarlos DV, *et al.* Randomized comparison of early versus late hyper-fractionated thoracic irradiation concurrently with chemotherapy in limited disease small-cell lung cancer: a randomized phase II study of the Hellenic Cooperative Oncology Group (HeCOG). Ann Oncol, 12: 1231–1238, 2001.

[24] Komaki R, Meyers CA, Shin DM, Garden AS, Byrne K, Nickens JA, Cox JD. Evaluation of cognitive function in patients with limited small cell lung cancer prior to and shortly following prophylactic cranial irradiation. Int J Rad Oncol Biol Phys, 33: 179–182, 1995.

[25] Gondi V, *et al.* Hippocampal-sparing whole-brain radiotherapy: a "how-to" technique using helical tomotherapy and linear accelerator–based intensity-modulated radiotherapy. Inter J Rad Oncology Biol Phys, 78: 1244–1252, 2010.

[26] NRG-CC003: A Randomized Phase II/III Trial of Prophylactic Cranial Irradiation with or without Hippocampal Avoidance for Small Cell Lung Cancer

[27] Langer CJ, Mehta, MP. Current management of brain metastases, with a focus on systemic options. J Clin Oncol, 23: 6207–6219, 2005.

[28] Russell A H, *et al.* Prophylactic cranial irradiation for lung cancer patients at high risk for development of cerebral metastasis: results of a prospective randomized trial conducted by the radiation therapy oncology group. Int J Rad Oncol Biol Phys, 21: 637–643, 1991.

[29] Gore EM, *et al.* Phase III comparison of prophylactic cranial irradiation versus observation in patients with locally advanced non-small-cell lung cancer: primary analysis of radiation therapy oncology group Study RTOG 0214. J Clin Oncol 29: 272–278, 2011.

[30] Sun A, *et al.* Phase III trial of prophylactic cranial irradiation compared with observation in patients with locally advanced non-small-cell lung cancer: neurocognitive and quality-of-life analysis. J Clin Oncol, 29: 279–286, 2011.

[31] Ettinger DS, *et al.* Non-small cell lung cancer, version 6. J Natl Compr Canc Netw, 13: 515–524, 2015.

[32] Gaspar L, *et al.* Recursive partitioning analysis (RPA) of prognostic factors in the radiation therapy oncology group (RTOG) brain metastases trials. Int J Rad Oncol Biol Phys, 37: 745–751, 1997.

http://dx.doi.org/10.5772/65869

[33] Sturm, V, *et al.* Stereotactic percutaneous single dose irradiation of brain metastases with a linear accelerator. Int J Rad Oncol Biol Phys, 13: 279–282, 1987.

[34] Aoyama H, Shirato H, Tago M, Nakagawa K, Toyoda T, Hatano K, Kenjyo M, Oya N, Hirota S, Shioura H, Kunieda E, Inomata T, Hayakawa K, Katoh N, Kobashi G. Stereotactic radiosurgery plus whole-brain radiation therapy *vs.* stereotactic radiosurgery alone for treatment of brain metastases: a randomized controlled trial. JAMA, 295: 2483-2491, 2006.

[35] Rekers, N, *et al.* Radiotherapy triggers durable immunotherapy responsiveness. Eur Soc Radiother Oncol, Abstr OC-234, 2016. Reviewed in Oncology Times, 38(17): 34, 2016.

Section 4

Status of Nanomedicine in Neurooncology

Chapter 4

Managing CNS Tumors: The Nanomedicine Approach

Juan Aparicio-Blanco and Ana-Isabel Torres-Suárez

Additional information is available at the end of the chapter

http://dx.doi.org/10.5772/66131

Abstract

Albeit the rapidly evolving knowledge about tumor biochemistry enables various new drug molecules to be designed as treatments, malignant central nervous system (CNS) tumors remain untreatable due to the failure to expose the entire tumor to such therapeutics at pharmacologically meaningful quantities. Therefore, drug delivery in CNS tumors must be properly addressed, as otherwise, novel therapies will continue to fail. In this regard, nanomedicine poses an appealing platform for efficient drug delivery to the CNS, since it may be targeted to improve the drug availability in the site of action, which would be translated into lower drug doses and fewer side effects. Hence, the accumulation of data about the CNS physiology and their relevant receptors, the widening therapeutic armamentarium of drugs potentially useful in CNS chemotherapy and the alternative routes for administration may envisage nanomedicines as a forthcoming routine approach. Indeed, on the basis of the promising results gathered from preclinical studies of nanomedicine-based therapy both systemically and locally administered, some nanomedicines have already been approved for clinical trials in a variety of CNS tumor conditions to serve as the first steps in the translation of nanotherapy to clinic. Their outcome will steer research directions for further improvements.

Keywords: central nervous system tumors, chemotherapy, brain targeting, clinical trials, local delivery, systemic delivery

1. Introduction

Primary central nervous system (CNS) tumors represent 2% of all cancers in adults, whereas this percentage increases to 15–25% in children. Primary brain tumors are stratified by the World Health Organization (WHO) according to a "malignancy scale". The WHO grade is closely related to clinical prognosis, ranging from grade I (with low proliferative potential and the possibility of cure following surgical resection alone) to grade IV (with widespread invasion of the surrounding healthy tissue, high proliferative potential, recurrence and fatal outcome). Unfortunately, many low-grade gliomas eventually often show progression to a higher histologic grade [1].

Gliomas represent approximately 80% of all malignant primary brain tumors. Glioblastomas (WHO grade IV) are the most frequent (54.4%) and aggressive type of glioma [2], although, in terms of treatment, WHO grade III brain tumors and glioblastomas are clustered together and treated similarly.

Although the management of brain tumors depends on the time of diagnosis, new onset or recurrence, the performance status and the age of the patient, the current standard approach in high-grade brain tumors combines maximal surgical resection (if eligible) with radiotherapy and concomitant and adjuvant chemotherapy as well as symptomatic treatment [3].

Available chemotherapy for high-grade brain tumors includes temozolomide, nitrosureas [carmustine (BCNU) and lomustine (CCNU)], topoisomerase inhibitors (etoposide, irinotecan), platinum agents (carboplatin), procarbazine, and vincristine. The first-line chemotherapy for newly diagnosed glioblastoma multiforme consists of temozolomide, whereas carmustine represents the second-line treatment. After the approval of temozolomide in 1999, irinotecan, etoposide, and platinum agents are mostly used only as adjuvant chemotherapy of bevacizumab (FDA approved in 2009 in monotherapy) for recurrent glioblastomas. In the case of WHO grade III gliomas (anaplastic astrocytomas and oligodendrogliomas), the first-line treatment is the PCV (procarbazine-lomustine-vincristine) combination [4].

Unfortunately, the efficacy of the treatment of brain tumors is questionable, since recurrence happens within 6.9 months of initial diagnosis. As a result, despite the combination of surgical resection, radiotherapy and concomitant temozolomide, glioblastoma multiforme remains incurable with a poor median survival of 14.6 months and 2-year survival rate of 26.5% [5]. This poor prognosis results from chemotherapy tumor resistance [6].

One of the chemoresistance mechanism best characterized relates to the expression of O^6-methylguanine-DNA methyltransferase (MGMT), a repair gene that removes alkyl groups from the O^6 position of guanine and consequently counteracts the alkylating agents (temozolomide or nitrosureas). Methylation of the promoter of this gene, which occurs in 35–45% of the cases, makes glioblastoma more sensitive to alkylating agents [7, 8].

Likewise, the existence of glioma stem cells greatly accounts for tumor recurrence, since they upregulate the expression level of P-gycoprotein [9], which is responsible for active efflux of many chemotherapy agents, including temozolomide.

The overexpression of epidermal growth factor receptor (EGFR), which ultimately triggers the activation of complex alternative signaling pathways, aimed at inhibiting apoptosis, also contributes to resistance to standard chemotherapy. Unfortunately, none of the receptor tyrosine kinase inhibitors and signal transduction inhibitors tested in clinical trials prolonged the mean survival, mainly due to the lack of successful drug delivery across the blood-brain tumor barrier (BBTB), since the exposure of the tumor to sublethal drug concentrations helps select the drug-resistant tumor cells [10].

The BBTB consists of the endothelium of existing and abnormal angiogenic blood vessels that deliver nutrients and oxygen to the tumor and enable widespread glioma migration to brain areas where the function of the barrier is still intact. Therefore, even though the BBTB is considered dysfunctional, the truth is that in low grade and in the infiltrative parts of high-grade gliomas, often responsible for the recurrence, the BBTB closely resembles the tight blood-brain barrier (BBB) typical of healthy brain capillaries [11]. Hence, the BBTB greatly accounts for the failure rate of the brain tumor therapy, since the hindrance to brain delivery of chemotherapeutic agents at pharmacologically effective levels conferred by this barrier cannot be offset by dose increase for fear of systemic toxicity. Furthermore, drug efflux pumps of the BBB can also be expressed in endothelium at the BBTB, representing an additional constraint to the achievement of adequate drug levels at the target site [12].

Since the therapeutic potential of chemotherapy greatly depends on its ability to attain pharmacologically effective levels at the entire diseased brain area, novel strategies to enhance drug delivery at the tumor site are strongly needed.

2. The nanomedicine approach

Conventional chemotherapy has failed to improve the prognosis of CNS tumors; hence novel drug delivery technologies have emerged under the assumption that targeted drug delivery could contribute to expose the entire tumor to therapeutically meaningful levels and ultimately improve treatment outcomes for brain tumors. An example of the success achievable thanks to advances in pharmaceutical technology is Gliadel®, the first FDA-approved brain cancer treatment to deliver chemotherapy directly to the tumor site in patients with malignant glioma for whom surgical resection is indicated. Gliadel® is a biodegradable wafer implanted on the surface of the resected tumor beds at the time of surgery that delivers carmustine steadily for about 3 weeks directly to the tumor site minimizing drug exposure to other areas of the body. Gliadel® contributes to eradicate the residual tumor cells at the resection margin and complements other standard therapies for brain tumors (surgery and radiotherapy) [13].

Nanomedicine represents an encouraging trend within the field of novel drug delivery technology with potential to preferentially delivering the drug at the target site and consequently overcoming biodistribution and pharmacokinetic limitations that eventually account for treatment failure of brain tumors. Nanomedicine is the application of nanotechnology in view of making a medical diagnosis or treating or preventing diseases. It exploits the improved and often novel properties of materials at a nanoscale. Nanomedicines are colloidal structures that act as drug carriers in which the drug substance is dissolved, entrapped, or encapsulated, or to which the drug substance is adsorbed or attached [14]. Unlike monolithic implants such as Gliadel®, colloidal carriers can be administered with conventional needles and therefore are not limited to those brain tumors where surgical resection is indicated.

Nanomedicine is especially relevant for chemotherapeutic agents, whose low dose availability at the tumor site cannot be counterbalanced by dose increase for fear of severe systemic side effects. Targeted nanomedicines would improve the availability of the drug at the scattered tumor bed and would allow obtaining therapeutic effects with lower drug doses and concomitantly minimizing the side effects of chemotherapy not only in unwanted peripheral tissues, but also in healthy brain cells. Therefore, the therapeutic index of drugs would be greatly enhanced thanks to nanomedicine. Targeted drug delivery to the site of action can be achieved through passive and active targeting or even through external physical stimuli. Passive targeting exploits the specific anatomical and functional features of the target tissues or cells to deliver drugs to the site of action. Active targeting requires the conjugation of tissue or cell-specific ligands on the surface of nanocarriers, whose recognition would eventually allow preferential accumulation of the drug at the diseased site. External stimuli such as a magnetic field, focused ultrasounds, light, and heat can also help selectively release the drug payload of nanomedicines at the target site [15].

Moreover, whereas most anticancer drugs are hydrophobic and often require to be solubilized in organic solvents for conventional administration, nanomedicines provide alternative formulations to administer chemotherapy without the need to use toxic solvents. Furthermore, nanomedicine is opening new therapeutic opportunities for easily degradable drug substances that cannot be used effectively as conventional formulations due to their short half-lives in vivo. Nanomedicines not only shield such drugs from enzymatic and chemical drug cleavage that accounts for the loss of pharmacological effect, but also can sustain and/or trigger drug release at a specific rate at the target site, resulting in maintenance of drug levels within a therapeutically desirable range. Thanks to this controlled release profile, undesirable pharmacokinetic properties of drug substances can be overcome with the use of nanocarriers and the dosing frequency can be improved to prescribe more comfortable dose regimens for patients.

The nanomedicine approach to enhance drug delivery to CNS tumors is highly versatile, since it would allow the coadministration of different anticancer agents and is compatible with both local and systemic routes of administration. In the current scenario, this approach must be directed toward surpassing acquired resistance to conventional chemotherapy and implementing strategies to boost the distribution across the brain endothelium in the case of systemic administration [16].

Nevertheless, nanomedicines might likewise cause unexpected toxicities as the other excipients also reach target tissues along with the drug. Nondegradable nanomedicines used for drug delivery would accumulate at the tumor site and would ultimately result in chronic inflammatory response, because, as colloidal systems, there is no chance of removing them after completion of the treatment. Albeit toxicity concerns of nanomedicines greatly rely on the relatively unexplored size-dependent properties and interaction with biological structures that strikingly differ from those of the bulk material, it is broadly agreed that the safety profile of brain-targeted nanomedicines would be improved with biocompatible excipients devoid of any short or long-term toxic effects [17]. Consequently, despite the large number of available biomaterials for nanomedicines preparation, only a few are suitable for brain tumor treatment because the CNS requires conservative choices with a proven track record of clinical safety. Nanomedicines developed for brain delivery mainly belong to three categories: polymer-based, lipid-based and metal-based, according to their major excipient (**Table 1**).

Category	Nanocarrier	Description	Size (nm)	Phase of development
Polymer-based	Polymeric nanoparticles	Solid matrix-like or reservoir-like nanostructures made up of biocompatible and biodegradable polymers or copolymers	20–1000	Preclinical
	Polymeric micelles	Nanostructures of amphiphilic diblock copolymers with a core of hydrophobic blocks stabilized by a corona of hydrophilic blocks	50–200	Preclinical
	Dendrimers	Highly branched tree-like nanostructures composed of a central core, internal branches, and reactive terminal groups	1–10	Preclinical
Lipid-based	Liposomes	Vesicles of amphipathic lipids structured in concentric bilayers surrounding an equal number of central aqueous compartments	80–200	Phase I, II clinical trials
	Solid lipid nanoparticles	Solid lipid matrixes at room and body temperatures that are stabilized by surfactant(s)	50–1000	Preclinical
	Lipid nanocapsules	Reservoir nanomedicines with a liquid oily core, surrounded by a shell of surfactants	20–100	Preclinical
Metal-based	Magnetic nanoparticles	Nanostructures composed of magnetic elements that can be manipulated using magnetic fields	10–50	Preclinical
	Gold nanoparticles	Nanostructures that can serve as drug carriers and even convert absorbed electromagnetic radiation to heat	5–50	Preclinical

Table 1. Main types of nanomedicines that are currently under investigation for the treatment of CNS tumors.

Overall, lipid-based nanomedicines may well be the most suitable for CNS drug delivery; insofar as lipids have very low toxicity, are biocompatible and biodegradable by nature, and the commercially available lipid-based formulations show a solid track record of clinical safety [18–20], whereas at present, only a few of the studied polymers for the development of polymer-based nanomedicines for brain drug delivery have demonstrated biocompatible, biodegradable, and nontoxic properties to be approved by the FDA for clinical use [21–23]. On the other hand, since the lack of biodegradation may not be appropriate for long-term administration, most metal-based nanomedicines (such as magnetic nanoparticles and gold nanoparticles) have been made more biocompatible and water-soluble with polymer coating [24].

3. Local delivery of nanomedicines

The local delivery of anticancer drugs serves to overcome the lack of specificity of conventional chemotherapy. Higher drug levels at the tumor site and lower drug distribution to healthy tissues account for the reduction of the systemic side effects with local routes of administration. Moreover, in the case of CNS tumors, local chemotherapy bypasses the major hurdle for systemic brain drug delivery: the blood-brain tumor barrier. However, the mechanical breach of this barrier may act as a double-edged sword since this might allow neurotoxic blood components to enter the brain or even enhance tumor dissemination.

Nanomedicines offer several advantages over conventional chemotherapy with regard to local CNS delivery: they can extend the exposure to short-brain-half-life drugs and provide long-lasting drug release that ultimately maintains therapeutic levels at the target site over longer periods. Moreover, nanomedicines show potential for enhancing antitumor activity via several pathways. First, locally administered nanomedicines can promote passive diffusion of the anticancer agent to the brain tumor tissue by increasing the local drug concentration gradient. Furthermore, nanomedicines can be actively targeted to the brain tumor cells by conjugating specific ligands that bind to the receptors that are overexpressed or uniquely expressed on the tumor surface (a mutant form of the epidermal growth factor receptor (EGFRvIII), interleukin receptors for interleukins 4 and 13) to efficiently trigger cellular uptake at the tumor site.

Similarly, locally administered nanomedicines can also help overcome some of the most troublesome chemoresistance mechanisms that are eventually responsible for tumor recurrence. In this sense, the upregulated expression of P-glycoprotein in drug-resistant cancer stem cells, which accounts for active efflux of most anticancer agents from the tumor area and reduces the effectiveness of chemotherapy, can be overcome thanks to nanomedicine. Indeed, the coating with nonionic surfactants seems to confer the nanocarrier itself with efflux-pump blockage properties [25]. Additionally, along with chemotherapy, nanomedicines can serve to deliver irreversible MGMT inhibitors (such as O^6-benzylguanine) and/or receptor tyrosine kinase inhibitors, to sensitize brain tumor cells to alkylating agents, and to counteract the inhibition of apoptosis mediated by the overexpression of the receptor of the epidermal growth factor (EGFR), respectively.

Several local routes of administration may be exploited by nanomedicines for handling of CNS tumors.

- The intracranial administration involves drug delivery directly into the brain parenchyma. Nonetheless, intraoperative infusion of anticancer drugs into brain tumors has experienced minor success given the diffusion-limited drug distribution, which does not allow the drug to reach the infiltrative area of recurrence. Moreover, the high interstitial fluid pressure and the presence of edema often observed in intracranial tumors may further hinder the diffusion of the infused agent.

Alternatively, convection-enhanced delivery (CED), another method for intracranial administration, achieves larger distribution volumes in the brain, for more homogeneous distribution within the tumor tissue, since it uses positive pressure to supplement simple diffusion with fluid convection. CED continuously delivers a bulk flow under a pressure gradient via a stereotactically guided catheter connected to a syringe pump. Drug leakage away from the tumor site [especially into the subarachnoid space with the subsequent drug spreading via the circulating cerebrospinal fluid (CSF)] should be avoided to minimize side effects such as chemical meningitis. In this regard, the suitable placement of catheters often prevents the leakage and helps spare healthy tissue.

CED can likewise deliver nanocarriers loaded with antineoplastic agents for CNS tumor therapy [26]. When combined with CED, the encapsulation of the drug infused into nanocarriers further reduces the potential side effects caused by drug leakage, while extends the brain half-life of anticancer agents by preventing them from being rapidly metabolized and/or eliminated by capillaries from the injection site. However, for efficient CED through the brain interstitium, the physicochemical properties of the colloidal systems must be optimized.

First, CED-injected nanomedicines must diffuse through interstitial spaces of the brain tissue. Hence, the size of the colloidal systems is a critical parameter to achieve optimal distribution volume with full coverage of the brain tumor tissue. Particles larger than 100 nm do not move readily through the brain interstitium, are retained near the administration site and do not distribute over clinically relevant volumes of brain tissue. Hence, in terms of size, the ideal nanocarrier for CED should be about 20–50 nm.

Moreover, to achieve optimal distribution volumes to cover both the tumor bed and the outlying cancer stem cells, it is convenient to provide nanocarriers with a hydrophilic coating [mostly polyethylene glycol (PEG) [27]]. The hydrophilic coating could help mask the hydrophobic structures, which would reduce the eventual binding to brain cells or to proteins in the interstitial space and ultimately enable greater diffusion. However, hydrophilic coating of nanocarriers also has the drawback of reducing the interactions with tumor cells, required for the loaded anticancer drug to eradicate the tumor. Alternatively, distribution volumes can be enhanced with the presence of co-infusates that serve to saturate the potential binding sites along the track of the infused nanomedicines. Furthermore, the ideal CED-administered nanocarrier should have a global neutral or negative charge to prevent nonspecific binding to negatively charged structures in the brain parenchyma and to achieve larger distribution volumes [27].

In addition, the infusion of viscous and hyperosmolar suspensions of nanocarriers would help reduce the risk of drug leakage and enhance the distribution volume by means of osmosis-mediated dilatation of the interstitial space through which nanocarriers could transit, respectively.

Nonetheless, despite its remarkable potential to improve clinical outcomes for CNS tumors, intracranial CED is an invasive neurosurgical procedure, which truly hinders its widespread use and limits the number of dosing cycles to be applied to eligible patients.

- The intrathecal administration involves the injection of anticancer drugs into the intrathecal space, which is the space that holds the cerebrospinal fluid (CSF). This can be achieved either with the implantation of an Ommaya reservoir (a dome-shaped container that is placed subcutaneously under the scalp during surgery, holds the chemotherapy and delivers it into the cerebral ventricles through a small catheter) or with direct injection into the CSF through a numbed area of the lower part of the spinal cord. Despite the significantly less invasive character of the second approach, intrathecal delivery fails to accumulate drugs in the brain parenchyma due to the bulk flow rate of CSF into the venous system, making this route optimal for the treatment of spinal tumors and disseminated meningeal metastases but not for parenchymal tumors like glioblastoma. Indeed, since meningeal gliomatosis remain protected by the blood-brain barrier, intrathecal delivery is widely considered a treatment approach for achieving improved outcomes for these patients [28].

Encapsulated drug	System	Model	Route of administration	References
Irinotecan	Liposomes	U87-bearing rats	CED	[30]
Irinotecan	Liposomes	GBM43-/SF7796-bearing mice	CED	[32]
Topotecan	Liposomes	U251-/U87MG-bearing rats	CED	[31, 36]
Topotecan + Doxorubicin	Liposomes	U87MG-bearing rats	CED	[33]
Irinotecan + Doxorubicin	Liposomes	U251-/U87MG-bearing rats	CED	[34]
Camptothecin	Polymer nanoparticles	9L-bearing rats	CED	[46]
Temozolomide	Polymer nanoparticles	U87-bearing rats	CED	[47]
HSVtk (+ intraperitoneal Ganciclovir)	Polymeric nanoparticles	9L-bearing rats	CED	[48]
Paclitaxel (+ radiotherapy)	Lipid nanocapsules	9L-bearing rats	CED	[49]
Ferrociphenol	Lipid nanocapsules	9L-bearing rats	CED	[37, 38, 50]
Ferrociphenol (+ radiotherapy)	Lipid nanocapsules	9L-bearing rats	CED	[51]
Metothrexate	Fifth-generation dendrimers	F98-bearing rats	CED	[42]
Cisplatin	Fifth-generation dendrimers	F98-bearing rats	CED	[43]
EGFRvIII antibody	Magnetic nanoparticles	U87 glioma-bearing mice	CED	[39]
Cetuximab	Magnetic nanoparticles	NO8-30, U87 and LN229-bearing mice	CED	[40]
O6-Benzylguanine (+ oral temozolomide)	Magnetic nanoparticles	GBM6-bearing mice	CED	[35]
Doxorubicin	Polymeric micelles	9L gliosarcoma-bearing rats	CED	[41]
Synthetic retinoid Am80 (+ intraperitoneal temozolomide)	Polymeric micelles	U87 glioma-bearing rats	CED	[52]
Camptothecin	Polymeric micelles	C6 glioma-bearing rats	Intranasal	[44]
Camptothecin + siRNA (Raf-1)	Polymeric micelles	C6 glioma-bearing rats	Intranasal	[45]

Table 2. Locally-administered nanomedicines already tested for efficacy in vivo against orthotopic rodent brain tumor models.

Unfortunately, not all anticancer agents are suitable for intrathecal delivery, as drug spread along the spinal canal can cause dose-limiting chemical arachoniditis. For those irritant drug substances, intrathecal delivery can take great advantage of nanomedicine, since their encapsulation into nanostructures could minimize drug exposure to toxic levels. As a proof of it, intrathecal-administered liposomal cytarabine (Depocyt®) has been approved for clinical use in lymphomatous meningitis. Nonetheless, the cytotoxicity of cytarabine against a wide spectrum of tumors makes Depocyt® a promising candidate for treating the above-mentioned forms of CNS cancer.

- More recently, the intranasal delivery has been proposed as an alternative local route of administration. Its noninvasive nature would allow self-administration by nasal inhalation and would enable the sterilization procedures of the drug dosage form to be avoided. This delivery route exploits the fact that trigeminal and olfactory nerves that innervate the nasal epithelium represent the only direct connection between the external environment and the brain [29]. However, this route appears to be relatively inefficient in delivering inhaled drugs to distant brain structures, mainly due to drug loss via systemic absorption.

In regard to brain tumor therapy, intranasal administration has received minor attention, with most applications of this approach being focused on the treatment of neurodegenerative diseases.

Numerous locally administered drug-loaded nanomedicines have already been assayed for efficacy in rodent models of brain tumors: liposomes, polymer nanoparticles, lipid nanocapsules, dendrimers, magnetic nanoparticles, and polymeric micelles, as summarized in **Table 2**. Although results are highly variable depending on various parameters, namely the tumor lineage and the onset, dose, and regimen of treatment, some general conclusions can be drawn from these preclinical studies. Overall, liposomes exhibited the most noticeable survival benefit and the presence of the highest percentage of long-term survivors [30, 31], partly because their potential as drug carriers was acknowledged earlier than any other alternative nanomedicine; hence research on nanomedicines for local CNS anticancer therapy has largely focused on liposomes.

Likewise, in some preclinical studies in rodent models, it was even evidenced that CED outperformed the survival benefit of the same formulation administered by a peripheral intravascular route [32]. Furthermore, the versatility of CED has enabled the coadministration of different liposomal formulations to enhance the effect of the anticancer agents [33, 34]. Concerning CED, numerous nanomedicines were formulated with a hydrophilic coating of polyethylene glycol and administered as slightly viscous suspensions to achieve optimal distribution volumes that cover the whole brain tumor tissue [35]. In fact, the deprivation of the hydrophilic coating, albeit increased median overall survival in comparison with untreated controls, significantly differed from efficacy findings reported for animals receiving the pegylated nanomedicines [36]. Nevertheless, it has been postulated the existence of a "threshold extent of pegylation," over which the hindrance conferred by polyethylene glycol to interact with the tumor cells counterbalances the increase in CED distribution volume provided by slight pegylation [37]. On the other hand, the addition of active targeting moieties that preferentially bind to receptors that are overexpressed on brain tumor cells to promote the delivery of nanomedicines to their target cells is controversial: whereas the attachment of OX26 or a cell-penetrating peptide has shown to enhance both tumor and healthy tissue internalization, which led to the appearance of side effects and high morbidity [38], the attachment of chlorotoxin or antibodies that selectively bind to the epidermal growth factor receptor mutant (EGFRvIII) present on human glioblastoma cells achieved significant survival benefits [35, 39, 40]. The different response could be explained by the choice of the ligand: ligands that preferentially bind to receptors on the cerebral endothelium are pointless in local delivery, whereas ligands that bind to receptors overexpressed on the brain tumor cells are those to be used for active targeting in local delivery.

Moreover, some studies [41–43] evidenced the importance of an adequate drug release to achieve a therapeutic response: the covalent linkage of methotrexate [42] and cisplatin [43] to dendrimer structures did not lead to any improvement in the median survival time of F98-bearing rats due to a release failure, while the survival benefit achieved with micellar doxorubicin in 9L-bearing rats was significantly relevant compared with CED of liposomal doxorubicin at the same dose due to the lack of release of doxorubicin from the liposomal formulation [41].

Importantly, CED-administered nanocarriers have been designed to overcome the MGMT-related chemoresistance to alkylating agents. O^6-benzylguanine has been loaded in iron oxide nanoparticles provided with a biocompatible chitosan-polyethylene glycol coating and actively targeted by chlorotoxin. The concurrent CED administration of these magnetic nanoparticles with oral temozolomide in mice implanted with a GBM6 clinically relevant xenograft extended by twofold the survival times in comparison with mice treated without the MGMT inhibitor and greatly mitigated the severe myelosuppression associated with systemic administration of free O^6-benzylguanine [35].

With regard to intranasal administration, polymeric micelles are the only nanomedicine type tested in rodent brain tumor models [44, 45]. The attachment of the cell-penetrating peptide Tat on their surface for actively enhancing the penetration rate across the nasal epithelium extended survival times [44].

4. Systemic delivery of nanomedicines

Thanks to the high brain perfusion rate, systemic intravascular administration is a very convenient strategy in the clinical management of cancer for compatibility with repeated drug administration and for its lower invasiveness in comparison with most local delivery routes. However, despite being considered disrupted to some extent, the presence of the BBTB has motivated the failure of conventional systemic chemotherapy for CNS tumors, since in low grade and along the infiltrating areas of high-grade gliomas where recurrences tend to occur, the BBTB closely resembles the nonfenestrated endothelial cells typical of healthy brain capillaries. Hence, the BBTB restricts the paracellular permeation of most anticancer agents into the CNS. As a result, conventional systemic chemotherapy must be administered at high drug doses, which causes severe dose-dependent side effects in healthy nontarget tissues.

Against this background of hindrance to brain tumor delivery, nanomedicine may enhance the distribution of poorly brain-distributed anticancer agents across the brain endothelium, since nanocarriers may well serve to target brain tumors through passive and active targeting or even through external physical stimuli [53]. Passive targeting occurs with the diffusion of nanomedicines through the interendothelial gaps of the highly vascularized leaky BBTB in the case of high-grade brain tumors, a phenomenon known as the enhanced retention and permeation (EPR) effect [54]. Moreover, surface-modified brain actively targeted nanomedicines may also enhance CNS delivery across the intact brain endothelium of infiltrative parts and low-grade brain tumors by triggering transcytosis either by ligand-receptor binding or by electrostatic interactions [55]. Therefore, nanomedicines can be useful for the treatment of different malignancy grades of brain tumors. In addition, the use of stimulus-sensitive groups to control drug release within the brain in a therapeutically relevant concentration could further enhance the specificity of the treatment effect to the brain tumor area. Alternatively, nanomedicines can block the active drug efflux back into the bloodstream.

For optimal passive targeting of brain tumors, systemic nanomedicines should have sufficient circulation time [56] to take advantage of the hypervascularized, leaky, and compromised lymphatic drainage system in a CNS tumor and selectively accumulate in the tumor tissue through the EPR effect. When given intravascularly, the larger the nanomedicines, the more susceptible to opsonization and removal by cells of the reticuloendothelial system (RES) [57]. Hence, to reduce opsonization in plasma and increase their plasma circulation time, the size of nanomedicines should be maintained below 100–200 nm. Additionally, the surface coating with hydrophilic polymers such as polyethylene glycol (PEG) to develop "stealth" nanomedicines creates a hydration layer that prevents protein adsorption and evades RES clearance [58], and consequently prolongs their circulation half-life.

Therefore, if properly designed, nanomedicines could cross the leaky BBTB in highly malignant brain tumors by passive targeting. Moreover, the BBTB can be artificially further disrupted to enable a wider distribution of nanomedicines to the brain tumor site. This disruption can be achieved via infusion of a hyperosmotic solution [59] or through the administration of vasoactive agents [60]. Hyperosmotic mannitol infusions cause a transient shrinkage of cerebrovascular endothelial cells, resulting in an enlargement of the tight junctions and BBTB leakiness. However, mannitol infusions also increase the permeability of healthy brain tissue, thereby increasing the risk of neurotoxicity. Conversely, the tumor vasculature is more sensitive than healthy brain vasculature to infusions with vasoactive agents (leukotrienes, bradykinin, and RMP-7, an analogue of bradykinin) through the transient activation of B2 receptors. Nevertheless, delivery of vasoactive agents requires intraarterial infusion, which increases the invasiveness of the procedure, and thereby creates a barrier for clinical translation of this approach. Alternatively, a local, transient, and reversible disruption of the BBTB can be generated by low-frequency focused ultrasound without permanent neuronal injury or other undesired long-term effects [61]. However, the artificial transient disruption of the BBTB is increasingly being considered undesirable since this might lead to widespread tumor dissemination and/or to the development of seizures due to the overexposure to neurotoxic blood components that enter the brain.

Additionally, optimal active targeting of nanomedicines would enable anticancer agents to be delivered across fully functional BBB of infiltrative areas and low-grade brain tumors exploiting carrier-mediated transportation, receptor-mediated, or adsorption-mediated transcytosis.

On the one hand, the carrier- and receptor-mediated active targeting involves functionalizing the surface of nanomedicines with moieties that specifically bind to receptors overexpressed on the brain endothelium and/or brain tumor cell membranes [62]. Therefore, different receptors in the brain could be employed:

- Penetration into the brain tumor area can be improved by simply targeting receptors that are normally overexpressed on the brain endothelium (such as transferrin receptors, nicotinic acetylcholine receptors, low-density lipoprotein receptor (LRP1), or carriers responsible for brain nutrient uptake) [62]. To target the transferrin receptor, both physiological ligands (transferrin and lactoferrin) and monoclonal antibodies (OX26 and 8D3) have been attached onto the surface of different types of nanomedicines [63–65]. Overall, physiological ligands ensure biocompatibility and nonimmunogenicity but develop competitive phenomena with endogenous ligands, whereas monoclonal antibodies prevent competitive phenomena with endogenous ligands since they bind to a different epitope. Likewise, nicotinic acetylcholine receptors have been targeted with peptides derived from snake neurotoxins, namely candoxin and Ophiophagushannah toxin b [66–68]. The peptide angiopep-2 has also been attached onto the surface of several nanomedicines to target LRP1 [69, 70]. Furthermore, glucose or mannose conjugation to nanomedicines has conferred brain-targeting properties through overexpressed facilitative glucose transporters [71, 72].

- Receptors distributed on proliferating endothelial cells in the tumor vasculature ($\alpha V\beta 3$ integrin, aminopeptidase N, nucleolin) represent additional potential sites for active targeting of nanomedicines to brain tumor tissue. In this sense, peptides containing the amino acid sequence Arg-Gly-Asp (RGD) have been coupled to the surface of distinct nanomedicines to bind to $\alpha V\beta 3$ integrin [73, 74]. Another tripeptide Asn-Gly-Arg (NGR) has been conjugated to different nanomedicines to target aminopeptidase N (CD 13) [75]. Moreover, the ability of the F3 peptide and the AS1411 aptamer to bind to nucleolin has been exploited to actively target nanomedicines to the brain tumor tissue [76, 77].

- Nanomedicines could also incorporate targeting moieties that bind to receptors that are overexpressed on tumor cells, to reduce the side effects of the antitumor agent on healthy brain cells after bypassing the BBTB. Apart from the already mentioned LRP1 and $\alpha V\beta 3$ integrin, these tumor targets include the receptor of the epidermal growth factor (EGFR) and its malignant isoform EGFRvIII, receptors for interleukins 13 (IL-13Rα2) and 4 (IL-4R), the folate and the insulin receptors, and even the membrane-bound matrix metalloproteinase-2 (MMP-2). Consequently, antibodies to EGFR or EGFRvIII have been conjugated to several nanomedicines for brain tumor targeting. Likewise, antiIL13Rα2 antibodies and IL-13 or IL-4-derived peptides (PEP-1 or AP-1, respectively) have been attached onto the surface of nanomedicines to selectively bind to interleukin receptors [78, 79]. To target the folate receptor, folid acid has been used, whereas to target the insulin receptor, the monoclonal antibody 83–14 has been incorporated to nanomedicines, since the use of the physiological ligand in this case was truly restricted by its biological effect on nontarget regions (namely hypoglycemia) [63]. Furthermore, MMP-2 has been widely targeted with nanomedicines coupled to a peptide derived from scorpion venom: chlorotoxin [65, 80].

Since any ligand for which a receptor exists on the cerebral endothelial or on the tumor cells might be used for active targeting, the enrichment of knowledge about the transport systems present on the BBB/BBTB and the glioma-specific receptors would enable novel practical approaches for improving the passage of nanomedicines to be designed with the purpose of exposing the entire diseased brain tumor area to pharmacologically meaningful quantities.

On the other hand, the adsorption-mediated active targeting takes advantage of electrostatic interactions between positively charged ligands and the negatively charged sialic acid residues in membrane glycoproteins of brain endothelial cells to trigger transcytosis. Hence, this type of active targeting involves modifying the surface of nanomedicines to make them positively charged, namely functionalization with cationic serum albumin and cell-penetrating peptides. The most frequently used cell-penetrating peptide for functionalization of nanomedicines is the transactivator of transcription peptide derived from HIV (TAT).

Subsequently, nanomedicines can also be designed to target simultaneously the BBB, the BBTB and the brain tumor cells by either attaching multiple targeting moieties, or by conjugating a single ligand that targets both the brain endothelia and the brain tumor cells [81]. In this case, nanomedicine could indeed represent a potential platform for targeting heterogeneous brain tumors [15].

Finally, nanomedicines can increase intratumoral concentration of systemically administered anticancer agents by inhibiting the efflux pump function of P-glycoprotein that is present at the BBTB and at the infiltrative tumor cells and that actively removes these drugs, accounting to a great extent for resistance to chemotherapy. A localized inhibition on brain efflux transporters can be achieved by co-loading pharmacological efflux pump inhibitors (such as tamoxifen) or by the nanomedicine itself, since the coating with nonionic surfactants seems to provide the nanocarrier itself with efflux-pump blockage properties.

Besides tailoring the size and surface properties of nanomedicines to influence intratumoral accumulation, external forces such as a magnetic field, light, and heat can also help selectively release the loaded drug of systemically administered nanomedicines at the tumor site [82]. Magnetic targeting has been applied under the assumption that magnetic nanoparticles can accumulate within a tumor area after systemic administration with a locally applied magnetic field. Another external force such as heat can be also used to control drug release in the case of nanomedicines whose excipients exhibit thermosensitive properties. Apart from enhancing tumor blood flow and vascular permeability, the application of local hyperthermia enables the drug to be easily released from thermosensitive nanomedicines when heating over the phase-transition temperature of the excipients.

Numerous intravenously administered drug-loaded nanomedicines have already been assayed for efficacy in rodent models of brain tumors: liposomes, polymer nanoparticles, lipid nanocapsules, dendrimers, polymeric micelles, magnetic nanoparticles, and gold nanoparticles (**Table 3**). Albeit results extremely depend on the tumor lineage and the onset, dose, and regimen of treatment, some general conclusions can be drawn. In broad terms, following intravenous administration, similar results were obtained with most types of nanomedicines.

Encapsulated drug	System	Strategy	Model	References
Paclitaxel	Liposomes	None	9L gliosarcoma-bearing rats	[89]
Paclitaxel	Liposomes	- Polyethylene glycol coating[a] - RGD peptide[b] - Histidine rich TH peptide[c]	C6 glioma-bearing mice	[73]
Irinotecan	Liposomes	- Polyethylene glycol coating[a]	U87MG glioblastoma-bearing mice	[90]
Topotecan	Liposomes	- Polyethylene glycol coating[a] - Wheat germ agglutinin[b] - Tamoxifen[d]	C6 glioma-bearing rats	[91]
Topotecan	Liposomes	- Polyethylene glycol coating[a]	U87M/GBM-43/GBM-6 glioblastoma-bearing mice	[92]
Doxorubicin	Liposomes	- Polyethylene glycol coating[a] - Folate[b] - Transferrin[b]	C6 glioma-bearing rats	[93]
Doxorubicin	Liposomes	- Lactoferrin[b] - Nanocarrier cationization[c]	C6 glioma-bearing rats	[94]
Doxorubicin	Liposomes	- Polyethylene glycol coating[a] - ^{D}CDX peptide[b]	U87MG glioblastoma-bearing mice	[66]
Doxorubicin	Liposomes	- Polyethylene glycol coating[a] - AP-1 peptide[b] - Focused ultrasound[e]	GBM8401 glioblastoma-bearing mice	[79]
Doxorubicin	Liposomes	- Polyethylene glycol coating[a] - Glutathione[b]	U87MG glioblastoma-bearing mice	[86]
Doxorubicin	Liposomes	- Polyethylene glycol coating[a] - Hyperthermia[e]	C6 glioma-bearing mice	[95]
Epirubicin	Liposomes	- Polyethylene glycol coating[a] - Transferrin[b] - Tamoxifen[d]	C6 glioma-bearing rats	[96]
Daunorubicin	Liposomes	- Polyethylene glycol coating[a] - Mannose[b] - Transferrin[b]	C6 glioma-bearing rats	[72]
RNA antiEGFR	Liposomes	- Polyethylene glycol coating[a] - 83-14[b] - 8D3[b]	U87MG glioblastoma-bearing mice	[63]
siRNA antiEGFR	Liposomes	- Polyethylene glycol coating[a] - T7 peptide[b]	U87MG glioblastoma-bearing mice	[64]
DNA (pC27)	Liposomes	- Polyethylene glycol coating[a] - OX26[b] - Chlorotoxine[b]	C6 glioma-bearing rats	[65]

http://dx.doi.org/10.5772/66131

Encapsulated drug	System	Strategy	Model	References
Paclitaxel	Polymeric nanoparticles	- Polyethylene glycol coating[a] - AS1411 aptamer[b]	C6 glioma-bearing rats	[77]
Paclitaxel	Polymeric nanoparticles	- Polyethylene glycol coating[a] - Peptide 22[b]	C6 glioma-bearing mice	[87]
Paclitaxel	Polymeric nanoparticles	- Polyethylene glycol coating[a] - F3 peptide[b]	C6 glioma-bearing mice	[76]
Paclitaxel	Polymeric nanoparticles	- Polyethylene glycol coating[a] - PEP-1[b]	C6 glioma-bearing mice	[97]
Paclitaxel	Polymeric nanoparticles	- Polyethylene glycol coating[a] - Glucose[b]	RG-2 glioma-bearing mice	[71]
Paclitaxel	Polymeric nanoparticles	- Polyethylene glycol coating[a] - APT peptide[b]	U87MG glioblastoma-bearing mice	[98]
Paclitaxel	Polymeric nanoparticles	- Polyethylene glycol coating[a] - iNGR peptide[b]	U87MG glioblastoma-bearing mice	[75]
Paclitaxel	Polymeric nanoparticles	- Polyethylene glycol coating[a] - RGD peptide[b]	U87MG glioblastoma-bearing mice	[74]
Paclitaxel	Polymeric nanoparticles	- Polyethylene glycol coating[a] - Angiopep[b]	U87MG glioblastoma-bearing mice	[70]
Gemcitabine	Polymeric nanoparticles	- Polysorbate-80 coating[a]	C6 glioma-bearing rats	[83]
Aclarubicin	Polymeric nanoparticles	- Polyethylene glycol coating[a] - Cationic serum albumin[c]	C6 glioma-bearing rats	[99]
Camptothecin	Polymeric nanoparticles	None	GL261 glioma-bearing mice	[84]
Doxorubicin	Polymeric nanoparticles	- Polysorbate-80 coating[a]	101-8 glioblastoma-bearing rats	[100]
Doxorubicin	Polymeric nanoparticles	- Polysorbate-80/Poloxamer-188/ Poloxamer-908 coating[a]	101-8 glioblastoma-bearing rats	[101]
Doxorubicin	Polymeric nanoparticles	- Polysorbate-80/Poloxamer-188 coating[a]	101-8 glioblastoma-bearing rats	[102]
Docetaxel	Polymeric nanoparticles	- Polyethylene glycol coating[a] - TGN peptide[b] - AS1411 aptamer[b]	C6 glioma-bearing mice	[78]
Docetaxel	Polymeric nanoparticles	- Polyethylene glycol coating[a] - IL-13 peptide[b]	U87MG glioblastoma-bearing mice	[103]
Porphyrin	Polymeric nanoparticles	- Polyethylene glycol coating[a] - F3 peptide[b] - Photodynamic therapy[e]	9L gliosarcoma-bearing rats	[104]

Encapsulated drug	System	Strategy	Model	References
Ferrociphenol	Lipid nanocapsules	- Polyethylene glycol coating[a]	9L gliosarcoma-bearing rats	[85]
Doxorubicin	Dendrimers	- Polyethylene glycol coating[a] - RGD peptide[b]	C6 glioma-bearing mice	[88]
RNA antiEGFR (miR-7)	Dendrimers	- Folate[b]	U251 glioma-bearing mice	[105]
DNA (TRAIL)	Dendrimers	- Polyethylene glycol coating[a] - Chlorotoxin[b]	C6 glioma-bearing mice	[80]
DNA (TRAIL)	Dendrimers	- Polyethylene glycol coating[a] - Angiopep[b]	C6 glioma-bearing mice	[69]
DNA (TRAIL)	Dendrimers	- Polyethylene glycol coating[a] - RGD peptide[b]	U87MG glioblastoma-bearing mice	[67]
Paclitaxel	Polymeric micelles	- Polyethylene glycol coating[a] - CDX peptide (candoxin)[b]		
Paclitaxel	Polymeric micelles	- Polyethylene glycol coating[a] - RGD peptide[b] - Transferrin[b]	U87MG glioblastoma-bearing mice	[106]
Paclitaxel	Polymeric micelles	- Polyethylene glycol coating[a] - KC2S peptide[b]	U87MG glioblastoma-bearing mice	[68]
Paclitaxel	Polymeric micelles	- Polyethylene glycol coating[a] - RGD peptide[b]	U87MG glioblastoma-bearing mice	[107]
Paclitaxel	Polymeric micelles	- Polyethylene glycol coating[a] - CDX peptide[b]	U87MG glioblastoma-bearing mice	[108]
Doxurubicin + Paclitaxel	Polymeric micelles	- Polyethylene glycol coating[a] - RGD peptide[b]	U87MG glioblastoma-bearing mice	[109]
SN-38 (camptothecin derivative)	Polymeric micelles	- Polyethylene glycol coating[a]	U87MG glioblastoma-bearing mice	[110, 111]
Paclitaxel	Magnetic nanoparticles	- Magnetic fields[e]	C6 glioma-bearing rats	[112]
Doxorubicin	Gold nanoparticles	- Polyethylene glycol coating[a] - TAT peptide[c]	U87MG glioblastoma-bearing mice	[113]

Strategies: [a]: passive targeting; [b]: carrier/receptor-mediated active targeting; [c]: adsorption-mediated active targeting; [d]: inhibition of efflux pump function; [e]: targeting caused by external physical stimuli

Table 3. Intravenously-administered nanomedicines already tested for efficacy in vivo against orthotopic rodent brain tumor models.

Most nanomedicines intended for preclinical evaluation following intravenous administration were designed to exploit passive and/or active targeting. Overall, stealth properties alone do not appear sufficient for enabling a nanoparticle-mediated transport into the brain, since in most cases of passively nonactively targeted nanomedicines survival benefits remained extremely modest [83–85].This could be due to the fact that PEG coating also reduces the tumor cell uptake of nanomedicines.

Additional active targeting using moieties that preferentially bind to receptors on the cerebral endothelial cells or overexpressed on brain tumor cells did indeed improve the therapeutic potential of nanomedicines due to preferential distribution to and within the brain tumor area: in all the studies with intravenously administered actively targeted nanomedicines, the median survival times were longer than their actively untargeted counterparts and noticeably longer than the untreated controls [75, 86–88].

However, most of these receptors are ubiquitously expressed to some degree. Hence, in order to prevent the occurrence of nonspecific side effects, dual-actively targeted have already been designed for achieving optimal targeting after systemic administration. In broad terms, the preclinical studies with these dual-targeted nanomedicines showed more extended survival times over their monotargeted counterparts [65, 73, 78].

5. Conclusions

Despite the tremendous efforts thus far, malignant CNS tumors still represent an unmet medical need. Albeit the rapidly evolving knowledge about tumor biochemistry enables various new drug molecules to be designed as treatments, drug delivery in CNS tumors deserves explicit attention, as otherwise, novel therapies will continue to fail to expose the entire tumor and the infiltrate cells that are not located in the tumor bed to such therapeutics at pharmacologically meaningful quantities. In this regard, nanomedicine poses an appealing platform for efficient drug delivery to the CNS, since it may be targeted to improve the availability of the drugs in their site of action, which could be translated into lower drug doses and fewer side effects.

The BBTB restricts the permeation of most anticancer agents into the CNS, especially in areas where the BBTB more closely resembles the BBB. Therefore, one major challenge in the field of systemic chemotherapy is the development of nanomedicines that can effectively overcome the BBTB and allow specific targeting of brain cancer cells. Overall, the features of nanomedicines dictate their biological fate: size and surface charge, the surface hydration and/or the presence of targeting ligands on the surface. Concerning brain endothelium permeation, an ideal systemic nanomedicine for CNS drug delivery should be around or smaller than 100 nm; be provided with a hydrophilic coating to avoid removal by the RES, extend its plasma half-life and indirectly increase the likelihood of crossing the brain endothelium; have targeting moieties to selectively enhance the distribution across the BBTB to the CNS and even be able to inhibit the drug efflux transporters at the BBTB.

ClinicalTrials.gov identifier	Condition	Treatment	Nanomedicine	Route of administration	Targeting approach	Phase
NCT00003073[u]	CNS tumors	Cytarabine	Liposome (DepoCyt®)	Intrathecal	None	I
NCT00029523[c]	Neoplastic meningitis	Cytarabine	Liposome (DepoCyt®)	Intrathecal	None	Unspecified
NCT00313599[c]	CNS tumors	Paclitaxel (+ oral lapatinib)	Albumin nanoparticles (Abraxane®)	Intravenous	None	I
NCT00019630[c]	Brain tumors (Children)	Doxorubicin	Pegylated liposome (Lipodox®)	Intravenous	Passive	I
NCT00465673[t]	Brain metastases	Doxorubicin	Pegylated liposome (Lipodox®)	Intravenous	Passive	II
NCT00734682[c]	Glioblastoma Gliosarcoma Anaplastic astrocytoma Anaplastic oligodendroglioma	Irinotecan	Pegylated liposome	Intravenous	Passive	I
NCT00854867[c]	Neoplastic meningitis	Cytarabine (+ concomitant/ sequential radiotherapy)	Liposome (DepoCyt®)	Intrathecal	None	I
NCT00944801[c]	Glioblastoma	Doxorubicin (+ temozolomide + radiotherapy)	Pegylated liposome (Caelix®)	Intravenous	Passive	I/II
NCT00964743[t]	Neoplastic meningitis	Cytarabine (+ oral sorafenib)	Liposome (DepoCyt®)	Intrathecal (Ommaya reservoir)	None	Unspecified
NCT00992602[c]	Leptomeningeal metastases	Cytarabine (+ intravenous methotrexate)	Liposome (DepoCyt®)	Intrathecal	None	II
NCT01044966[t]	Glioblastoma multiforme Glioma Astrocytoma Brain tumor	Cytarabine (+ oral temozolomide)	Liposome (DepoCyt®)	Intrathecal	None	I/II
NCT01222780[c]	Brain tumors (Children)	Vincristine	Liposome (Marqibo®)	Intravenous	None	I/II
NCT01386580[c]	Recurrent malignant glioma Brain metastases	Doxorubicin	Glutathione pegylated liposome	Intravenous	Passive + Active	I/II

http://dx.doi.org/10.5772/66131

ClinicalTrials.gov identifier	Condition	Treatment	Nanomedicine	Route of administration	Targeting approach	Phase
NCT01563614[t]	Leptomeningeal metastases	Cytarabine (+ oral lomustine + radiotherapy)	Liposome (DepoCyt®)	Intrathecal	None	I
NCT01818713[u]	Leptomeningeal metastases	Doxorubicin	Glutathione pegylated liposome	Intravenous	Passive + Active	II
NCT02022644[r]	High-grade glioma	Irinotecan	Pegylated liposome	CED	Passive	I
NCT02340156[r]	Glioblastoma	Normal human wild type p53 DNA sequence (+ oral temozolomide)	Anti-transferrin receptor single-chain antibody cationic liposome	Intravenous	Active	II

Identifier of the current state of the clinical trial: [u]: unknown; [c]: completed; [t]: terminated; [r]: recruiting.

Table 4. Nanomedicines that have already reached the clinical trials stage for the treatment of CNS tumors.

Alternatively, nanomedicines can be locally administered to bypass the BBTB. However, CED and intrathecal delivery remain invasive approaches that carry significant risks for patients. An optimal nanomedicine for CED should be below 100 nm, neutral or negatively charged, conjugated to specific ligands that bind the tumor cell receptors and be infused in a slight viscous and hyperosmolar solution.

Overall, nanomedicines intended for brain delivery either for systemic or local delivery should ideally be biocompatible and biodegradable, have a controllable release profile to trigger drug release at the site of action, be able to be sterilized and have a feasible industrial production for clinical implementation.

On the basis of the promising results gathered from preclinical studies of nanomedicine-based therapy, some nanomedicines have already been approved for clinical trials in a variety of CNS tumors conditions to serve as the first steps in translation of nanotherapy to clinic (**Table 4**). Therefore, their outcome will steer further research directions and when successful, will provide handles for further improvements. Unfortunately, the results of the already completed clinical trials are not yet available on clinicaltrials.gov.

It is worth underlining the fact that current clinical trials using nanomedicines for brain tumors are conducted on patients who have failed conventional therapy and have very poor prognosis (mostly recurrent high-grade glioma or brain metastases). However, expanding the application of nanomedicine to less aggressive forms of brain cancer is challenging, as long as the long-term side effects due to the interactions of colloids with biological structures are not yet known and, consequently, the regulatory agencies have not yet developed comprehensive regulatory guidelines for nanomedicines.

In view of the approved clinical trials, some general conclusions can be drawn. On the one hand, whereas several liposomal formulations are already under clinical trials, the rest of types of nanomedicines are lagging behind. The investigation of nanomedicines for CNS delivery has focused largely on liposomal preparations mostly due to the fact that their potential as drug carriers was already acknowledged back in the 1970s, much earlier than any other alternative nanocarrier.

On the other hand, most liposomes that reached clinical trials for the treatment of brain tumors are passively targeted, avoiding the ligand-receptor interaction. Despite the promising preclinical results, translation of active targeting to clinical trials poses some challenges, since most targeted receptors are not exclusively present at the BBTB and/or brain tumor cells, which may give raise to side effects. Additionally, nanomedicines conjugated with physiological ligands can develop competitive phenomena with endogenous ligands and dysregulate their homeostasis, whereas nanomedicines that incorporate monoclonal antibodies must be able to interact with human receptors to not cause immunogenic reactions; hence, presumably different from those antibodies assayed in rodent preclinical models. Nonetheless, two actively targeted liposomes have recently made their way to clinical trials to cross the BBB after intravenous injection for achieving higher and efficacious brain drug levels: 2B3-101 is a PEGylated liposomal doxorubicin formulation conjugated with glutathione and SGT-53 is a cationic liposome conjugated with an antitransferrin receptor single-chain antibody and encapsulating a normal human wild-type p53 DNA sequence to restore the wild-type p53 function and downmodulate MGMT activity in order to increase the sensitivity of tumor cells to alkylating agents.

Concerning the different routes of administration, intravenous among the systemic routes and CED and intrathecal delivery among the local routes have even made its way into clinical trials for nanoparticle administration.

In conclusion, clinical implementation of nanomedicines for patients with brain tumors is still in its infancy. However, further clinical studies of brain-targeted nanomedicines are warranted in the future, with increasing incidences of CNS cancers, many of whom being terrible rapidly progressing and so far untreatable tumors. Hence, the accumulation of data about the CNS physiology and about relevant receptors, the widening therapeutic armamentarium of drugs potentially useful in CNS chemotherapy, the alternative routes for administration and the estimation of the brain permeability with in vitro BBB models to early triage the potential of nanomedicines for optimum therapy of brain tumors envisage nanomedicines as a forthcoming routine approach [114].

Acknowledgements

This work was partially funded by the Research Group GR35/10 Santander-UCM, Group: Parenteral Administration of Drugs. Juan Aparicio-Blanco thanks the Spanish Ministry of Education for the Contract within the Professor Training Program FPU (Ref. FPU13/02325).

http://dx.doi.org/10.5772/66131

Author details

Juan Aparicio-Blanco and Ana-Isabel Torres-Suárez*

*Address all correspondence to: galaaaa@ucm.es

Department of Pharmaceutical Technology, Faculty of Pharmacy, Complutense University, Madrid, Spain

References

[1] Louis DN, Ohgaki H, Wiestler OD, Cavenee WK, Burger PC, Jouvet A, Scheithauer BW, Kleihues P. The 2007 WHO classification of tumours of the central nervous system. Acta Neuropathol. 2007;114:97–109.

[2] Schwartzbaum JA, Fisher JL, Aldape KD, Wrensch M. Epidemiology and molecular pathology of glioma. Nat Clin Pract Neurol. 2006;2:494–503.

[3] Wen PY, Kesari S. Malignant gliomas in adults. N Engl J Med. 2008;359:492–507.

[4] Alifieris C, Trafalis DT. Glioblastoma multiforme: pathogenesis and treatment. Pharmacol Ther. 2015;152:63–82.

[5] Stupp R, Mason WP, van den Bent MJ, Weller M, Fisher B, Taphoorn MJB, Belanger K, Brandes AA, Marosi C, Bogdahn U, Curschmann J, Janzer RC, Ludwin SK, Gorlia T, Allgeier A, Lacombe D, Cairncross JG, Eisenhauer E, Mirimanoff RO, Van Den Weyngaert D, Kaendler S, Krauseneck P, Vinolas N, Villa S, Wurm RE, Maillot MHB, Spagnolli F, Kantor G, Malhaire JP, Renard L, De Witte O, Scandolaro L, Vecht CJ, Maingon P, Lutterbach J, Kobierska A, Bolla M, Souchon R, Mitine C, Tzuk-Shina T, Kuten A, Haferkamp G, de Greve J, Priou F, Menten J, Rutten I, Clavere P, Malmstrom A, Jancar B, Newlands E, Pigott K, Twijnstra A, Chinot O, Reni M, Boiardi A, Fabbro M, Campone M, Bozzino J, Frenay M, Gijtenbeek J, Brandes AA, Delattre JY, Bogdahn U, De Paula U, van den Bent MJ, Hanzen C, Pavanato G, Schraub S, Pfeffer R, Soffietti R, Weller M, Kortmann RD, Taphoorn M, Torrecilla JL, Marosi C, Grisold W, Huget P, Forsyth P, Fulton D, Kirby S, Wong R, Fenton D, Fisher B, Cairncross G, Whitlock P, Belanger K, Burdette-Radoux S, Gertler S, Saunders S, Laing K, Siddiqui J, Martin LA, Gulavita S, Perry J, Mason W, Thiessen B, Pai H, Alam ZY, Eisenstat D, Mingrone W, Hofer S, Pesce G, Curschmann J, Dietrich PY, Stupp R, Mirimanoff RO, Thum P, Baumert B, Ryan G, European Org Res Treatment Canc B. Radiotherapy plus concomitant and adjuvant temozolomide for glioblastoma. N Engl J Med. 2005;352:987–996.

[6] Messaoudi K, Clavreul A, Lagarce F. Toward an effective strategy in glioblastoma treatment. Part I: resistance mechanisms and strategies to overcome resistance of glioblastoma to temozolomide. Drug Discov Today. 2015;20:899–905.

[7] Esteller M, Garcia-Foncillas J, Andion E, Goodman SN, Hidalgo OF, Vanaclocha V, Baylin SB, Herman JG. Inactivation of the DNA-repair gene MGMT and the clinical response of gliomas to alkylating agents. N Engl J Med. 2000;343:1350–1354.

[8] Hegi ME, Diserens A, Gorlia T, Hamou M, de Tribolet N, Weller M, Kros JM, Hainfellner JA, Mason W, Mariani L, Bromberg JEC, Hau P, Mirimanoff RO, Cairncross JG, Janzer RC, Stupp R. MGMT gene silencing and benefit from temozolomide in glioblastoma. N Engl J Med. 2005;352:997–1003.

[9] de Faria GP, de Oliveira JA, de Oliveira JGP, Romano SD, Neto VM, Maia RC. Differences in the expression pattern of P-glycoprotein and MRP1 in low-grade and high-grade gliomas. Cancer Invest. 2008;26:883–889.

[10] Holohan C, Van Schaeybroeck S, Longley DB, Johnston PG. Cancer drug resistance: an evolving paradigm. Nat Rev Cancer. 2013;13:714–726.

[11] VanTellingen O, Yetkin-Arik B, De Gooijer MC, Wesseling P, Wurdinger T, De Vries HE. Overcoming the blood-brain tumor barrier for effective glioblastoma treatment. Drug Resist Update. 2015;19:1–12.

[12] Schinkel AH. P-glycoprotein, a gatekeeper in the blood-brain barrier. Adv Drug Deliv Rev. 1999;36:179–194.

[13] Westphal M, Hilt DC, Bortey E, Delavault P, Olivares R, Warnke PC, Whittle IR, Jaaskelainen J, Ram Z. A phase 3 trial of local chemotherapy with biodegradable carmustine (BCNU) wafers (Gliadel wafers) in patients with primary malignant glioma. Neuro-Oncology. 2003;5:79–88.

[14] Davis ME, Chen Z, Shin DM. Nanoparticle therapeutics: an emerging treatment modality for cancer. Nat Rev Drug Discov. 2008;7:771–782.

[15] Cheng Y, Morshed RA, Auffinger B, Tobias AL, Lesniak MS. Multifunctional nanoparticles for brain tumor imaging and therapy. Adv Drug Deliv Rev. 2014;66:42–57.

[16] Karim R, Palazzo C, Evrard B, Piel G. Nanocarriers for the treatment of glioblastoma multiforme: current state-of-the-art. J Control Release. 2016;227:23–37.

[17] Cupaioli FA, Zucca FA, Boraschi D, Zecca L. Engineered nanoparticles. How brain friendly is this new guest? Prog Neurobiol. 2014;119:20–38.

[18] Lai F, Fadda AM, Sinico C. Liposomes for brain delivery. Expert Opin Drug Deliv. 2013;10:1003–1022.

[19] Gastaldi L, Battaglia L, Peira E, Chirio D, Muntoni E, Solazzi I, Gallarate M, Dosio F. Solid lipid nanoparticles as vehicles of drugs to the brain: current state of the art. Eur J PharmBiopharm. 2014;87:433–444.

[20] Aparicio-Blanco J, Torres-Suarez AI. Glioblastoma multiforme and lipid nanocapsules: a review. J Biomed Nanotechnol. 2015;11:1283–1311.

[21] Patel T, Zhou JB, Piepmeier JM, Saltzman WM. Polymeric nanoparticles for drug delivery to the central nervous system. Adv Drug Deliv Rev. 2012;64:701–705.

[22] Costantino L, Boraschi D. Is there a clinical future for polymeric nanoparticles as brain-targeting drug delivery agents? Drug Discov Today. 2012;17:367–378.

[23] Mishra V, Kesharwani P. Dendrimer technologies for brain tumor. Drug Discov Today. 2016;21:766–778.

[24] Singh D, McMillan JM, Kabanov AV, Sokolsky-Papkov M, Gendelman HE. Bench-to-bedside translation of magnetic nanoparticles. Nanomedicine. 2014;9:501–516.

[25] Jabr-Milane LS, van Vlerken LE, Yadav S, Amiji MM. Multi-functional nanocarriers to overcome tumor drug resistance. Cancer Treat Rev. 2008;34:592–602.

[26] Allard E, Passirani C, Benoit JP. Convection-enhanced delivery of nanocarriers for the treatment of brain tumors. Biomaterials. 2009;30:2302–2318.

[27] MacKay JA, Deen DF, Szoka FC. Distribution in brain of liposomes after convection enhanced delivery; modulation by particle charge, particle diameter, and presence of steric coating. Brain Res. 2005;1035:139–153.

[28] Serwer LP, James CD. Challenges in drug delivery to tumors of the central nervous system: an overview of pharmacological and surgical considerations. Adv Drug Deliv Rev. 2012;64:590–597.

[29] Mistry A, Stolnik S, Illum L. Nanoparticles for direct nose-to-brain delivery of drugs. Int J Pharm. 2009;379:146–157.

[30] Noble CO, Krauze MT, Drummond DC, Yamashita Y, Saito R, Berger MS, Kirpotin DB, Bankiewicz KS, Park JW. Novel nanoliposomal CPT-11 infused by convection-enhanced delivery in intracranial tumors: pharmacology and efficacy. Cancer Res. 2006;66:2801–2806.

[31] Saito R, Krauze MT, Noble CO, Drummond DC, Kirpotin DB, Berger MS, Park JW, Bankiewicz KS. Convection-enhanced delivery of Ls-TPT enables an effective, continuous, low-dose chemotherapy against malignant glioma xenograft model. Neuro-Oncology. 2006;8:205–214.

[32] Chen PY, Ozawa T, Drummond DC, Kalra A, Fitzgerald JB, Kirpotin DB, Wei KC, Butowski N, Prados MD, Berger MS, Forsayeth JR, Bankiewicz K, James CD. Comparing routes of delivery for nanoliposomal irinotecan shows superior anti-tumor activity of local administration in treating intracranial glioblastoma xenografts. Neuro-Oncology. 2013;15:189–197.

[33] Yamashita Y, T Krauze M, Kawaguchi T, Noble CO, Drummond DC, Park JW, Bankiewicz KS. Convection-enhanced delivery of a topoisomerase I inhibitor (nanoliposomaltopotecan) and a topoisomerase II inhibitor (pegylated liposomal doxorubicin) in intracranial brain tumor xenografts. Neuro-Oncology. 2007;9:20–28.

[34] Krauze MT, Noble CO, Kawaguchi T, Drummond D, Kirpotin DB, Yamashita Y, Kullberg E, Forsayeth J, Park JW, Bankiewicz KS. Convection-enhanced delivery of nanoliposomal CPT-11 (irinotecan) and PEGylated liposomal doxorubicin (Doxil) in rodent intracranial brain tumor xenografts. Neuro-Oncology. 2007;9:393–403.

[35] Stephen ZR, Kievit FM, Veiseh O, Chiarelli PA, Fang C, Wang K, Hatzinger SJ, Ellenbogen RG, Silber JR, Zhang MQ. Redox-responsive magnetic nanoparticle for targeted convection-enhanced delivery of o-6-benzylguanine to brain tumors. ACS Nano. 2014;8:10383–10395.

[36] Grahn AY, Bankiewicz KS, Dugich-Djordjevic M, Bringas JR, Hadaczek P, Johnson GA, Eastman S, Luz M. Non-PEGylated liposomes for convection-enhanced delivery of topotecan and gadodiamide in malignant glioma: initial experience. J Neuro-Oncol. 2009;95:185–197.

[37] Huynh NT, Passirani C, Allard-Vannier E, Lemaire L, Roux J, Garcion E, Vessieres A, Benoit JP. Administration-dependent efficacy of ferrociphenol lipid nanocapsules for the treatment of intracranial 9L rat gliosarcoma. Int J Pharm. 2012;423:55–62.

[38] Laine AL, Huynh NT, Clavreul A, Balzeau J, Bejaud J, Vessieres A, Benoit JP, Eyer J, Passirani C. Brain tumour targeting strategies via coated ferrociphenol lipid nanocapsules. Eur J Pharm Biopharm. 2012;81:690–693.

[39] Hadjipanayis CG, Machaidze R, Kaluzova M, Wang LY, Schuette AJ, Chen HW, Wu XY, Mao H. EGFRvIII antibody-conjugated Iron Oxide nanoparticles for magnetic resonance imaging-guided convection-enhanced delivery and targeted therapy of glioblastoma. Cancer Res. 2010;70:6303–6312.

[40] Kaluzova M, Bouras A, Machaidze R, Hadjipanayis CG. Targeted therapy of glioblastoma stem-like cells and tumor non-stem cells using cetuximab-conjugated iron-oxide nanoparticles. Oncotarget. 2015;6:8788–9806.

[41] Inoue T, Yamashita Y, Nishihara M, Sugiyama S, Sonoda Y, Kumabe T, Yokoyama M, Tominaga T. Therapeutic efficacy of a polymeric micellar doxorubicin infused by convection-enhanced delivery against intracranial 9L brain tumor models. Neuro-Oncology. 2009;11:151–157.

[42] Wu G, Barth RF, Yang WL, Kawabata S, Zhang LW, Green-Church K. Targeted delivery of methotrexate to epidermal growth factor receptor-positive brain tumors by means of cetuximab (IMC-C225) dendrimer bioconjugates. Mol Cancer Ther. 2006;5:52–59.

[43] Barth RF, Wu G, Meisen WH, Nakkula RJ, Yang W, Huo T, Kellough DA, Kaumaya P, Turro C, Agius LM, Kaur B. Design, synthesis, and evaluation of cisplatin-containing EGFR targeting bioconjugates as potential therapeutic agents for brain tumors. Onco Targets Ther. 2016;9:2769–2781.

[44] Taki H, Kanazawa T, Akiyama F, Takashima Y, Okada H. Intranasal delivery of camptothecin-loaded tat-modified nanomicells for treatment of intracranial brain tumors. Pharmaceuticals (Basel, Switzerland). 2012;5:1092–1102.

[45] Kanazawa T, Morisaki K, Suzuki S, Takashima Y. Prolongation of life in rats with malignant glioma by intranasal siRNA/drug codelivery to the brain with cell-penetrating peptide-modified micelles. Mol Pharm. 2014;11:1471–1478.

[46] Sawyer AJ, Saucier-Sawyer JK, Booth CJ, Liu J, Patel T, Piepmeier JM, Saltzman WM. Convection-enhanced delivery of camptothecin-loaded polymer nanoparticles for treatment of intracranial tumors. Drug Deliv Transl Res. 2011;1:34–42.

[47] Bernal GM, LaRiviere MJ, Mansour N, Pytel P, Cahill KE, Voce DJ, Kang SJ, Spretz R, Welp U, Noriega SE, Nunez L, Larsen G, Weichselbaum RR, Yamini B. Convection-enhanced delivery and in vivo imaging of polymeric nanoparticles for the treatment of malignant glioma. Nanomed-Nanotechnol Biol Med. 2014;10:149–157.

[48] Mangraviti A, Tzeng SY, Kozielski KL, Wang Y, Jin YK, Gullotti D, Pedone M, Buaron N, Liu A, Wilson DR, Hansen SK, Rodriguez FJ, Gao GD, DiMeco F, Brem H, Olivi A, Tyler B, Green JJ. Polymeric nanoparticles for nonviral gene therapy extend brain tumor survival in vivo. ACS Nano. 2015;9:1236–1249.

[49] Vinchon-Petit S, Jarnet D, Paillard A, Benoit JP, Garcion E, Menei P. In vivo evaluation of intracellular drug-nanocarriers infused into intracranial tumours by convection-enhanced delivery: distribution and radiosensitisation efficacy. J Neuro-Oncol. 2010;97:195–205.

[50] Allard E, Huynh NT, Vessieres A, Pigeon P, Jaouen G, Benoit JP, Passirani C. Dose effect activity of ferrocifen-loaded lipid nanocapsules on a 9L-glioma model. Int J Pharm. 2009;379:317–323.

[51] Allard E, Jarnet D, Vessieres A, Vinchon-Petit S, Jaouen G, Benoit JP, Passirani C. Local delivery of Ferrociphenol Lipid nanocapsules followed by external Radiotherapy as a synergistic treatment against intracranial 9L glioma xenograft. Pharm Res. 2010;27:56–64.

[52] Yokosawa M, Sonoda Y, Sugiyama S, Saito R, Yamashita Y, Nishihara M, Satoh T, Kumabe T, Yokoyama M, Tominaga T. Convection-enhanced delivery of a synthetic retinoid Am80, loaded into polymeric micelles, prolongs the survival of rats bearing intracranial glioblastoma xenografts. Tohoku J Exp Med. 2010;221:257–264.

[53] Peluffo H, Unzueta U, Negro-Demontel ML, Xu ZK, Vaquez E, Ferrer-Miralles N, Villaverde A. BBB-targeting, protein-based nanomedicines for drug and nucleic acid delivery to the CNS. Biotechnol Adv. 2015;33:277–287.

[54] Maeda H, Wu J, Sawa T, Matsumura Y, Hori K. Tumor vascular permeability and the EPR effect in macromolecular therapeutics: a review. J Control Release. 2000;65:271–284.

[55] Beduneau A, Saulnier P, Benoit JP. Active targeting of brain tumors using nanocarriers. Biomaterials. 2007;28:4947–4967.

[56] Alyautdin R, Khalin I, Nafeeza MI, Haron MH, Kuznetsov D. Nanoscale drug delivery systems and the blood-brain barrier. Int J Nanomed. 2014;9:795–811.

[57] Dobrovolskaia MA, McNeil SE. Immunological properties of engineered nanomaterials. Nat Nanotechnol. 2007;2:469–478.

[58] Gref R, Luck M, Quellec P, Marchand M, Dellacherie E, Harnisch S, Blunk T, Muller RH. 'Stealth' corona-core nanoparticles surface modified by polyethylene glycol (PEG): influences of the corona (PEG chain length and surface density) and of the core composition on phagocytic uptake and plasma protein adsorption. Colloid Surf B-Biointerfaces. 2000;18:301–313.

[59] Rapoport SI, Robinson PJ. Tight-junctional modification as the basis of osmotic opening of the blood-brain barrier. Ann NY Acad Sci. 1986;481:250–267.

[60] Nakano S, Matsukado K, Black KL. Increased brain tumor microvessel permeability after intracarotid bradykinin infusion is mediated by nitric oxide. Cancer Res. 1996;56:4027–4031.

[61] Hynynen K, McDannold N, Vykhodtseva N, Raymond S, Weissleder R, Jolesz FA, Sheikov N. Focal disruption of the blood-brain barrier due to 260-kHz ultrasound bursts: a method for molecular imaging and targeted drug delivery. J Neurosurg. 2006;105:445–454.

[62] Oller-Salvia B, Sanchez-Navarro M, Giralt E, Teixido M. Blood-brain barrier shuttle peptides: an emerging paradigm for brain delivery. Chemical Society Reviews. 2016;45:4690–4707.

[63] Zhang Y, Zhang YF, Bryant J, Charles A, Boado RJ, Pardridge WM. Intravenous RNA interference gene therapy targeting the human epidermal growth factor receptor prolongs survival in intracranial brain cancer. Clin Cancer Res. 2004;10:3667–3677.

[64] Wei L, Guo X-Y, Yang T, Yu M-Z, Chen D-W, Wang J-C. Brain tumor-targeted therapy by systemic delivery of siRNA with Transferrin receptor-mediated core-shell nanoparticles. Int J Pharm. 2016;510:394–405.

[65] Yue PJ, He L, Qiu SW, Li Y, Liao YJ, Li XP, Xie D, Peng Y. OX26/CTX-conjugated PEGylated liposome as a dual-targeting gene delivery system for brain glioma. Mol Cancer. 2014;13:13.

[66] Wei XL, Zhan CY, Shen Q, Fu W, Xie C, Gao J, Peng CM, Zheng P, Lu WY. A D-Peptide ligand of Nicotine Acetylcholine Receptors for brain-targeted drug delivery. Angew Chem-Int Edit. 2015;54:3023–3027.

[67] Zhan CY, Wei XL, Qian J, Feng LL, Zhu JH, Lu WY. Co-delivery of TRAIL gene enhances the anti-glioblastoma effect of paclitaxel in vitro and in vivo. J Control Release. 2012;160:630–636.

[68] Zhan CY, Yan ZQ, Xie C, Lu WY. Loop 2 of Ophiophagushannah Toxin b binds with Neuronal Nicotinic Acetylcholine receptors and enhances intracranial drug delivery. Mol Pharm. 2010;7:1940–1947.

[69] Huang SX, Li JF, Han L, Liu SH, Ma HJ, Huang RQ, Jiang C. Dual targeting effect of Angiopep-2-modified, DNA-loaded nanoparticles for glioma. Biomaterials. 2011;32: 6832–6838.

[70] Xin HL, Sha XY, Jiang XY, Zhang W, Chen LC, Fang XL. Anti-glioblastoma efficacy and safety of paclitaxel-loading Angiopep-conjugated dual targeting PEG-PCL nanoparticles. Biomaterials. 2012;33:8167–8176.

[71] Jiang XY, Xin HL, Ren QY, Gu JJ, Zhu LJ, Du FY, Feng CL, Xie YK, Sha XY, Fang XL. Nanoparticles of 2-deoxy-D-glucose functionalized poly(ethylene glycol)-co-poly(trimethylene carbonate) for dual-targeted drug delivery in glioma treatment. Biomaterials. 2014;35:518–529.

[72] Ying X, Wen H, Lu WL, Du J, Guo J, Tian W, Men Y, Zhang Y, Li RJ, Yang TY, Shang DW, Lou JN, Zhang LR, Zhang Q. Dual-targeting daunorubicin liposomes improve the therapeutic efficacy of brain glioma in animals. J Control Release. 2010;141:183–192.

[73] Shi KR, Long Y, Xu CQ, Wang Y, Qiu Y, Yu QW, Liu YY, Zhang QY, Gao HL, Zhang ZR, He Q. Liposomes combined an integrin alpha(v)beta(3)-specific vector with pH-responsible cell-penetrating property for highly effective antiglioma therapy through the blood-brain barrier. ACS Appl Mater Interfaces. 2015;7:21442–1454.

[74] Jiang XY, Sha XY, Xin HL, Xu XM, Gu JJ, Xia WY, Chen S, Xie YK, Chen LC, Chen YZ, Fang XL. Integrin-facilitated transcytosis for enhanced penetration of advanced gliomas by poly(trimethylene carbonate)-based nanoparticles encapsulating paclitaxel. Biomaterials. 2013;34:2969–2979.

[75] Kang T, Gao XL, Hu QY, Jiang D, Feng XY, Zhang X, Song QX, Yao L, Huang M, Jiang XG, Pang ZQ, Chen HZ, Chen J. iNGR-modified PEG-PLGA nanoparticles that recognize tumor vasculature and penetrate gliomas. Biomaterials. 2014;35:4319–4332.

[76] Hu QY, Gu GZ, Liu ZY, Jiang MY, Kang T, Miao DY, Tu YF, Pang ZQ, Song QX, Yao L, Xia HM, Chen HZ, Jiang XG, Gao XL, Chen J. F3 peptide-functionalized PEG-PLA nanoparticles co-administrated with tLyp-1 peptide for anti-glioma drug delivery. Biomaterials. 2013;34:1135–1145.

[77] Guo JW, Gao XL, Su LN, Xia HM, Gu GZ, Pang ZQ, Jiang XG, Yao L, Chen J, Chen HZ. Aptamer-functionalized PEG-PLGA nanoparticles for enhanced anti-glioma drug delivery. Biomaterials. 2011;32:8010–8020.

[78] Gao HL, Qian J, Cao SJ, Yang Z, Pang ZQ, Pan SQ, Fan L, Xi ZJ, Jiang XG, Zhang QZ. Precise glioma targeting of and penetration by aptamer and peptide dual-functioned nanoparticles. Biomaterials. 2012;33:5115–5123.

[79] Yang FY, Wong TT, Teng MC, Liu RS, Lu M, Liang HF, Wei MC. Focused ultrasound and interleukin-4 receptor-targeted liposomal doxorubicin for enhanced targeted drug delivery and antitumor effect in glioblastoma multiforme. J Control Release. 2012;160:652–658.

[80] Huang RQ, Ke WL, Han LA, Li JF, Liu SH, Jiang C. Targeted delivery of chlorotoxin-modified DNA-loaded nanoparticles to glioma via intravenous administration. Biomaterials. 2011;32:2399–2406.

[81] Liu Y, Lu WY. Recent advances in brain tumor-targeted nano-drug delivery systems. Expert Opin Drug Deliv. 2012;9:671–686.

[82] Liu HL, Hua MY, Yang HW, Huang CY, Chu PC, Wu JS, Tseng IC, Wang JJ, Yen TC, Chen PY, Wei KC. Magnetic resonance monitoring of focused ultrasound/magnetic nanoparticle targeting delivery of therapeutic agents to the brain. Proc Natl AcadSci U S A. 2010;107:15205–15210.

[83] Wang CX, Huang LS, Hou LB, Jiang L, Yan ZT, Wang YL, Chen ZL. Antitumor effects of polysorbate-80 coated gemcitabine polybutylcyanoacrylate nanoparticles in vitro and its pharmacodynamics in vivo on C6 glioma cells of a brain tumor model. Brain Res. 2009;1261:91–99.

[84] Householder KT, DiPerna DM, Chung EP, Wohlleb GM, Dhruv HD, Berens ME, Sirianni RW. Intravenous delivery of camptothecin-loaded PLGA nanoparticles for the treatment of intracranial glioma. Int J Pharm. 2015;479:374–380.

[85] Huynh NT, Morille M, Bejaud J, Legras P, Vessieres A, Jaouen G, Benoit JP, Passirani C. Treatment of 9L gliosarcoma in rats by Ferrociphenol-loaded lipid nanocapsules based on a passive targeting strategy via the EPR effect. Pharm Res. 2011;28:3189–3198.

[86] Gaillard PJ, Appeldoorn CCM, Dorland R, van Kregten J, Manca F, Vugts DJ, Windhorst B, van Dongen G, de Vries HE, Maussang D, Van Tellingen O. Pharmacokinetics, brain delivery, and efficacy in brain tumor-bearing mice of glutathione pegylated liposomal doxorubicin (2B3–101). PLoS One. 2014;9:10.

[87] Zhang B, Sun XY, Mei H, Wang Y, Liao ZW, Chen J, Zhang QZ, Hu Y, Pang ZQ, Jiang XG. LDLR-mediated peptide-22-conjugated nanoparticles for dual-targeting therapy of brain glioma. Biomaterials. 2013;34:9171–9182.

[88] Zhang LH, Zhu SJ, Qian LL, Pei YY, Qiu YM, Jiang YY. RGD-modified PEG-PAMAM-DOX conjugates: In vitro and in vivo studies for glioma. Eur J Pharm Biopharm. 2011;79:232–240.

[89] Zhou R, Mazurchuk RV, Tamburlin JH, Harrold JM, Mager DE, Straubinger RM. Differential pharmacodynamic effects of paclitaxel formulations in an intracranial rat brain tumor model. J Pharmacol Exp Ther. 2010;332:479–488.

[90] Noble CO, Krauze MT, Drummond DC, Forsayeth J, Hayes ME, Beyer J, Hadaczek P, Berger MS, Kirpotin DB, Bankiewicz KS, Park JW. Pharmacokinetics, tumor accumulation and antitumor activity of nanoliposomal irinotecan following systemic treatment of intracranial tumors. Nanomedicine. 2014;9:2099–2108.

[91] Du J, Lu WL, Ying X, Liu Y, Du P, Tian W, Men Y, Guo J, Zhang Y, Li RJ, Zhou J, Lou JN, Wang JC, Zhang X, Zhang Q. Dual-targeting topotecan liposomes modified with tamoxifen and wheat germ agglutinin significantly improve drug transport across the

blood-brain barrier and survival of brain tumor-bearing animals. Mol Pharm. 2009;6:905–917.

[92] Serwer LP, Noble CO, Michaud K, Drummond DC, Kirpotin DB, Ozawa T, Prados MD, Park JW, James CD. Investigation of intravenous delivery of nanoliposomaltopotecan for activity against orthotopic glioblastoma xenografts. Neuro-Oncology. 2011;13:1288–1295.

[93] Gao JQ, Lv Q, Li LM, Tang XJ, Li FZ, Hu YL, Han M. Glioma targeting and blood-brain barrier penetration by dual-targeting doxorubincin liposomes. Biomaterials. 2013;34:5628–5639.

[94] Chen HL, Qin Y, Zhang QY, Jiang W, Tang L, Liu J, He Q. Lactoferrin modified doxorubicin-loaded procationic liposomes for the treatment of gliomas. Eur J Pharm Sci. 2011;44:164–173.

[95] Gong W, Wang ZY, Liu N, Lin W, Wang XP, Xu D, Liu HY, Zeng CY, Xie XY, Mei XG, Lu WL. Improving efficiency of adriamycin crossing blood brain barrier by combination of thermosensitive liposomes and hyperthermia. Biol Pharm Bull. 2011;34:1058–1064.

[96] Tian W, Ying X, Du J, Guo J, Men Y, Zhang Y, Li RJ, Yao HJ, Lou JN, Zhang LR, Lu WL. Enhanced efficacy of functionalized epirubicin liposomes in treating brain glioma-bearing rats. Eur J Pharm Sci. 2010;41:232–243.

[97] Wang BY, Lv LY, Wang Z, Jiang Y, Lv W, Liu X, Wang ZY, Zhao Y, Xin HL, Xu QW. Improved anti-glioblastoma efficacy by IL-13R alpha 2 mediated copolymer nanoparticles loaded with paclitaxel. Sci Rep. 2015;5:13.

[98] Gu GZ, Hu QY, Feng XY, Gao XL, Jiang ML, Kang T, Jiang D, Song QX, Chen HZ, Chen J. PEG-PLA nanoparticles modified with APT(EDB) peptide for enhanced anti-angiogenic and anti-glioma therapy. Biomaterials. 2014;35:8215–8226.

[99] Lu W, Wan J, Zhang Q, She ZJ, Jiang XG. Aclarubicin-loaded cationic albumin-conjugated pegylated nanoparticle for glioma chemotherapy in rats. Int J Cancer. 2007;120:420–431.

[100] Steiniger SCJ, Kreuter J, Khalansky AS, Skidan IN, Bobruskin AI, Smirnova ZS, Severin SE, Uhl R, Kock M, Geiger KD, Gelperina SE. Chemotherapy of glioblastoma in rats using doxorubicin-loaded nanoparticles. Int J Cancer. 2004;109:759–767.

[101] Ambruosi A, Gelperina S, Khalansky A, Tanski S, Theisen A, Kreuter J. Influence of surfactants, polymer and doxorubicin loading on the anti-tumour effect of poly(butyl cyanoacrylate) nanoparticles in a rat glioma model. J Microencapsul. 2006;23:582–592.

[102] Gelperina S, Maksimenko O, Khalansky A, Vanchugova L, Shipulo E, Abbasova K, Berdiev R, Wohlfart S, Chepurnova N, Kreuter J. Drug delivery to the brain using surfactant-coated poly(lactide-co-glycolide) nanoparticles: influence of the formulation parameters. Eur J Pharm Biopharm. 2010;74:157–163.

[103] Gao HL, Yang Z, Zhang S, Cao SJ, Shen S, Pang ZQ, Jiang XG. Ligand modified nanoparticles increases cell uptake, alters endocytosis and elevates glioma distribution and internalization. Sci Rep. 2013;3:8.

[104] Reddy GR, Bhojani MS, McConville P, Moody J, Moffat BA, Hall DE, Kim G, Koo YEL, Woolliscroft MJ, Sugai JV, Johnson TD, Philbert MA, Kopelman R, Rehemtulla A, Ross BD. Vascular targeted nanoparticles for imaging and treatment of brain tumors. Clin Cancer Res. 2006;12:6677–6686.

[105] Liu XZ, Li G, Su ZG, Jiang ZM, Chen L, Wang JF, Yu SZ, Liu ZL. Poly(amido amine) is an ideal carrier of miR-7 for enhancing gene silencing effects on the EGFR pathway in U251 glioma cells. Oncol Rep. 2013;29:1387–1394.

[106] Zhang PC, Hu LJ, Yin Q, Feng LY, Li YP. Transferrin-modified c RGDfK -paclitaxel loaded hybrid micelle for sequential blood-brain barrier penetration and glioma targeting therapy. Mol Pharm. 2012;9:1590–1598.

[107] Zhan CY, Gu B, Xie C, Li J, Liu Y, Lu WY. Cyclic RGD conjugated poly(ethylene glycol)-co-poly(lactic acid) micelle enhances paclitaxel anti-glioblastoma effect. J Control Release. 2010;143:136–142.

[108] Zhan CY, Li B, Hu LJ, Wei XL, Feng LY, Fu W, Lu WY. Micelle-based brain-targeted drug delivery enabled by a nicotine acetylcholine receptor ligand. Angew Chem-Int Edit. 2011;50:5482–5485.

[109] Huang YK, Liu WC, Gao F, Fang XL, Chen YZ. c(RGDyK)-decorated pluronic micelles for enhanced doxorubicin and paclitaxel delivery to brain glioma. Int J Nanomed. 2016;11:1629–1641.

[110] Kuroda JI, Kuratsu JI, Yasunaga M, Koga Y, Saito Y, Matsumura Y. Potent antitumor effect of SN-38-incorporating polymeric micelle, NK012, against malignant glioma. Int J Cancer. 2009;124:2505–2511.

[111] Kuroda J, Kuratsu J, Yasunaga M, Koga Y, Kenmotsu H, Sugino T, Matsumura Y. Antitumor effect of NK012, a 7-ethyl-10-hydroxycamptothecin-Incorporating polymeric micelle, on U87MG orthotopic glioblastoma in mice compared with irinotecan hydrochloride in combination with bevacizumab. Clin Cancer Res. 2010;16:521–529.

[112] Zhao M, Liang C, Li AM, Chang J, Wang HJ, Yan RM, Zhang JJ, Tai JL. Magnetic paclitaxel nanoparticles inhibit glioma growth and improve the survival of rats bearing glioma xenografts. Anticancer Res. 2010;30:2217–2223.

[113] Cheng Y, Dai Q, Morshed RA, Fan XB, Wegscheid ML, Wainwright DA, Han Y, Zhang LJ, Auffinger B, Tobias AL, Rincon E, Thaci B, Ahmed AU, Warnke PC, He C, Lesniak MS. Blood-brain barrier permeable gold nanoparticles: an efficient delivery platform for enhanced malignant glioma therapy and imaging. Small. 2014;10:5137–5150.

[114] Aparicio-Blanco J, Martin-Sabroso C, Torres-Suarez A-I. In vitro screening of nanomedicines through the blood brain barrier: a critical review. Biomaterials. 2016;103:229–255.

Section 5

CNS Malignancies and Genetic Association

Chapter 5

Phakomatoses and Their Tumors: Genetics and New Treatment Options

Muhammad Taimur Malik,
Mohammed Faraz Majeed and Scott G. Turner

Additional information is available at the end of the chapter

http://dx.doi.org/10.5772/66207

Abstract

In addition to sporadic primary neoplasms of the central nervous system, several genetic syndromes associated with CNS tumors have been identified. Tuberous sclerosis, neurofibromatosis-1 and -2, and von Hippel–Lindau syndrome belong to a collection of disorders called phakomatoses, which include both CNS tumors and cutaneous manifestations. The underlying genetics of these disorders are being elucidated and offer novel therapies for intervention.

Keywords: genetic, phakomatosis, tuberous sclerosis, neurofibromatosis, von Hippel–Lindau

1. Introduction

Phakomatoses are disorders which, in addition to skin manifestations, can lead to the development of tumors within the central and peripheral nervous systems. Due to extensive organ involvement and the complex genetics pathways involved, treatment options are limited. Some of these genetic disorders involve abnormal neural crest migration or terminal differentiation, and tumor suppressor gene dysfunction. These may exhibit autosomal dominant or X-linked recessive inheritance.

Central nervous system manifestations include seizure, stroke, hearing loss secondary to tumor growth, visual loss secondary to optic gliomas, hydrocephalus, and cognitive deficits, while peripheral manifestations include sensory loss or motor weakness from neurofibromas. The cutaneous manifestations of these disorders are usually ectodermal in origin and can and range from small lesions to involvement of entire dermatomes. The common disorders leading to tumor development are tuberous sclerosis, neurofibromatosis-1 and -2, and von Hippel–Lindau syndrome. Ataxia-telangiectasia and Sturge–Weber syndrome are phakomatoses that do not typically lead to tumor development and will not be discussed here.

2. Tuberous sclerosis

2.1. Introduction

Tuberous sclerosis complex (TSC) is a disorder affecting 1:5000–1:10,000 live births [1] characterized by the formation of hamartomas throughout the brain and skin with the formation of renal, pulmonary, and cardiac tumors [2]. It is thought to be caused by mutations in two genes: TSC1on chromosome 9q34 encoding hamartin [3] and TSC2 on chromosome 16p13 encoding tuberin [4]. These mutations result in varying degrees of upregulation of the mTOR pathway. About 10–15% of TSC patients do not have mutations in TSC1 or TSC2, however. While often inherited in an autosomal dominant fashion, two-thirds of patients have de novo mutations [5].

Patients most often present in the first year of life with seizures, typically focal seizures or infantile spasms. The latter are closely associated with cognitive impairments but they typically respond to vigabatrin [6]. A spectrum of cognitive, behavioral, neuropsychiatric, and intellectual disabilities has been described known as TSC-associated neuropsychiatric disorders (TAND), for which there is currently inadequate screening and no approved treatment [7]. Within the brain are found tubers within the cortex and subependymal nodules (SEN) along the walls of the lateral and third ventricles. SEN may transform into subependymal giant cell astrocytomas (SEGA). Retinal astrocytic hamartomas occur in 30–50% of TSC patients and most remain stable over time. They are typically asymptomatic unless they involve the macula or optic nerve [8].

Approximately, 55–80% of patients with TSC have renal involvement including renal cysts, polycystic kidney disease (PKD), and angiomyolipomas (AML) [9]. The Polycystin-1 gene (PKD-1), mutations in which lead to polycystic kidney disease, is downstream of TSC2 and a TSC2/PKD1 contiguous gene syndrome has been described in which deletions affecting both genes lead to TSC with early-onset renal polycystic disease [10]. AML are benign tumors with components of abnormal blood vessels, immature smooth muscle, and mature adipose tissue. They are often multiple, bilateral, and grow mainly during childhood, remaining relatively stable in adulthood [11]. They are associated with an increased risk of micro- and macroaneurysms [12]. Sequelae of the renal manifestations of TSC include an increased risk of hemorrhage from abnormal vasculature, chronic kidney disease, and hypertension.

In TSC, cardiac rhabdomyomas occur, which are more common in neonates and may spontaneously regress throughout childhood. They occur in 20% of adults with TSC. Most are asymptomatic, though arrhythmias including Wolff-Parkinson-White syndrome or outflow obstruction may occur, warranting treatment [13].

Lymphangioleiomyomatosis is an uncommon progressive cystic lung disease affecting 30% of women and a milder form in 10% of men with TSC, associated with mutations in

http://dx.doi.org/10.5772/66207

the TSC2 gene. Abnormal smooth muscle cells proliferate and infiltrate into alveoli, blood vessels, and lymphatics causing obstructive airway disease and blood vessel and lymphatic obstruction leading to dyspnea, pneumothorax, and chylous pleural effusion [14].

The neurocutaneous manifestations of TSC are present in over 90% of patients and include hypomelanotic macules (87–100%), shagreen patches (20–80%), ungual fibromas (17–87%), and angiofibromas (47–90%) [15].

2.2. Diagnosis

The pathogenesis of TSC is thought to be due in part to changes in neural crest function. Neural crest cells arise from embryonic ectoderm and give rise to a number of diverse cell lineages including melanocytes. Cutaneous lesions, particularly hypomelanotic macules and shagreen patches, are due in part to abnormal segmental melanocytic distribution and the characteristic dermal facial angiofibromas are derived from mesencephalic neural crest. Cortical tubers and hamartomas in the periventricular region and are not neural crest derivatives, however [16].

Cortical tubers are developmental in origin and histologically show effacement of the laminar architecture with gliosis, micro-calcifications, large multinucleated cells with glassy, bright eosinophilic cytoplasm, and dysmorphic neurons. These neurons appear "immature" with poorly differentiated cell processes, abundant eosinophilic cytoplasm, and disrupted orientation within the cortical lamina. These structures are believed to be responsible for seizures in TSC patients [17]. Subependymal nodules (SEN) are neoplasms that develop along the walls of the lateral ventricles and can calcify within the first few years of life. These may subsequently develop into subependymal giant cell astrocytoma [18].

SEGA typically develop from SEN in the first two decades of life and present clinically with worsening epilepsy or increased intracranial pressure from obstructive hydrocephalus. These mixed glioneural tumors tend to be well-circumscribed with a variety of tumor cell morphologies including large pleomorphic, multinucleated gemistocytic astrocytes, and small, spindle-shaped astrocytes as well as giant ganglionic pyramidal cells (**Figure 1**). Perivascular pseudorosettes and calcifications are commonly seen. These benign tumors have a low (1–7%) mitotic index and correspond to WHO grade I. Immunohistochemistry demonstrates immunoreactivity for both glial (S-100 and GFAP) and neural (neurofilament, class III β-tubulin, and synaptophysin) markers, again emphasizing the divergent glioneuronal origin of these tumors [19]. Because the ependyma remains intact over SEGA, dissemination of tumor cells into the CSF is rare.

Radiographically, cortical tubers appear as areas of increased cortical and subcortical intensity on T2-weighted magnetic resonance imaging (MRI) and rarely enhance with gadolinium [20]. In contrast, cerebellar tubers are usually wedge-shaped and distort the architecture of the folia. Up to half are calcified and may enhance with gadolinium. They are not epileptogenic and can change in size or enhancement over the first decade of life. Subependymal nodules are T1 hyper-intense and T2 hypo-intense lesions along the lateral ventricles that often enhance with gadolinium and are described as having the appearance of "candle drip-

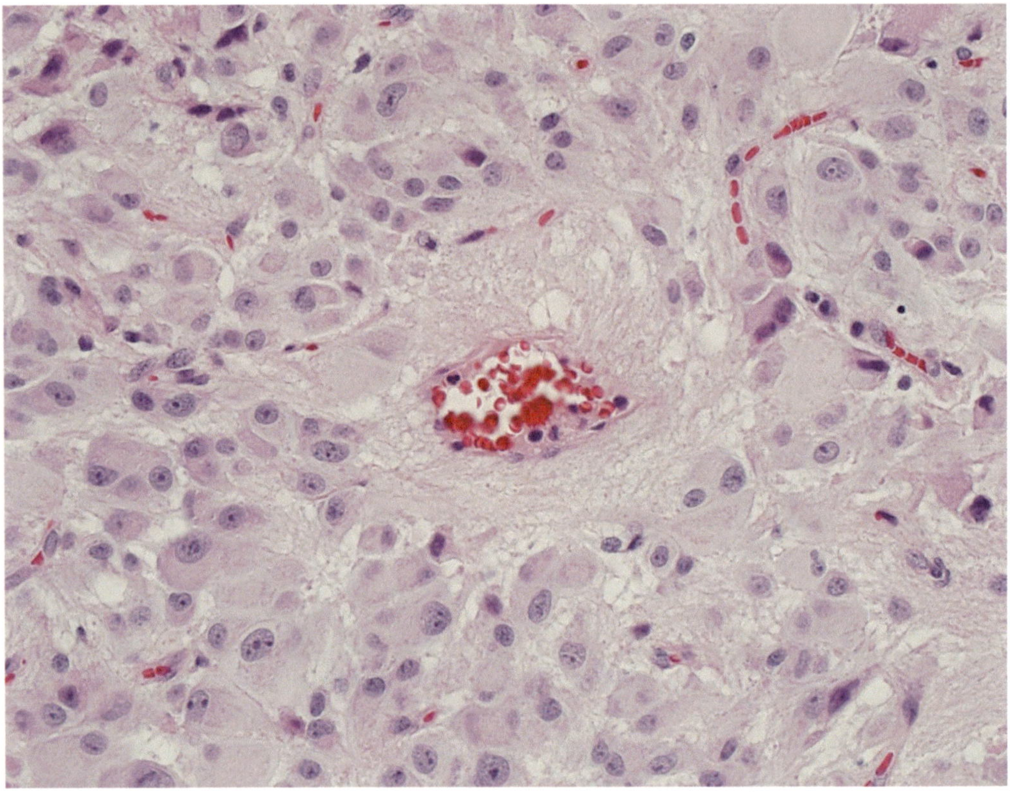

Figure 1. SEGA histology: large cells with abundant cytoplasm and prominent nucleoli, and a perivascular fibrillary area.

pings" [21]. SEGA appear as round to ovoid lesions that are iso- to hypo-intense on T1 MRI and hyper-intense on T2 MRI. They often avidly enhance with gadolinium and calcification and hemorrhage may be seen (**Figure 2**). In addition, radial migration lines may be seen on FLAIR images that represent gliosis resulting from aberrant glial neuronal migration [22].

2.3. Genetics

Mutations in two genes have been identified that lead to TSC. TSC1 on chromosome 9q34 encodes a 130 kDa protein called hamartin and TSC2 on chromosome 16p13 encodes the 200 kDa protein tuberin. TSC2 mutations are more common and are associated with a more severe phenotype [2]. These two proteins form a heterodimeric complex that integrates signals from various pathways involved in regulating cellular responses to environmental stress and energy status (**Figure 3**). TSC2 contains a GTP-activating domain (GAP) that has been shown to activate the small GTPase Rheb [23], which in turn activates mechanistic target of rapamycin complex-1 (mTORC1). mTORC1 is a serine-threonine protein kinase complex whose activation leads to cell growth and differentiation by inhibiting autophagy and promoting protein and lipid synthesis through the phosphatidylinositol 3-kinase-related kinase signaling pathway [24]. TSC1 has no catalytic function and serves to stabilize TSC2 [25].

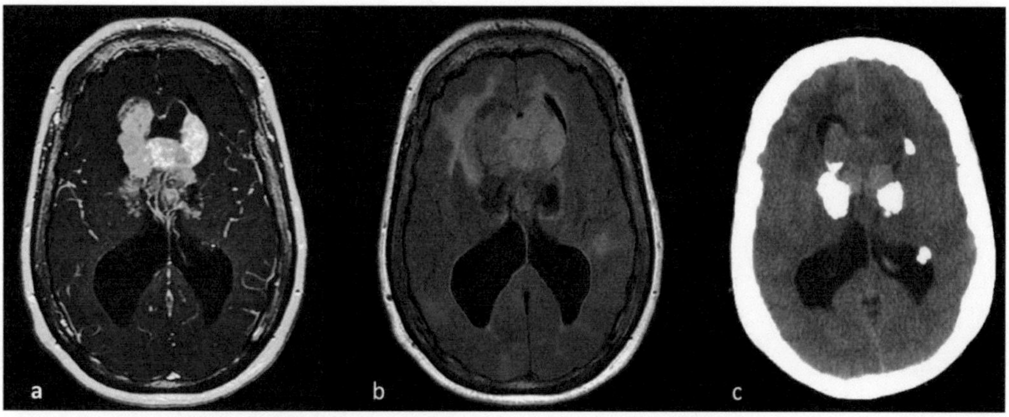

Figure 2. Subependymal Giant Cell Asrocytoma: (a) MRI axial T1 with gadolinium (b) MRI axial T2 FLAIR (c) Head CT showing prominent calcification.

TSC1/2 is regulated by a number of factors. Many growth factors and cytokines act through AKT (protein kinase B), which inhibits TSC1/2 by phosphorylating TSC2 ([26]. Ribosomal S6 kinase (RSK) activates extracellular signal-regulated kinase (ERK), which then phosphorylates and inactivates TSC2. RSK also directly phosphorylates TSC2 [27]. A number of environmental cues lead to TSC1/TSC2 activation. Environmental stress leading to low ATP/AMP ratio leads to activation of AMP-dependent protein kinase (AMPK) that phosphorylates and activates TSC2. Hypoxia induces expression of hypoxia-inducible factor-α (HIF1α) that induces REDD1, which indirectly activates TSC1-TSC2 by removing AKT dependent inhibition [28].

The mTOR1 complex (mTORC1) is a multimeric complex consisting of deptor, PRAS40, raptor, mLST8, mTOR, and TTI1–TEL and effects changes in several important cellular processes [24]. mTORC1 promotes protein synthesis through activation of the translation initiation promoter S6K and through inhibition of the inhibitory mRNA cap binding 4E-BP1. This pathway is thought to play a role in formation of hamartomas. mTORC1 inhibits autophagy through inhibitory phosphorylation of ULK1, preventing formation of the ULK1–ATG13–FIP200 complex required for initiation of autophagy [29]. Increased mTORC1 signaling may cause hypopigmented macules by affecting autophagy during melanogenesis.

Recently, TBC1D7 has been identified as a third subunit in the TSC1/TSC2 complex. This protein does not seem to reflect changes in cellular growth conditions, but loss of TBC1D7 leads to destabilization of TSC1/TSC2 and decreased Rheb-GAP activity [30].

2.4. Treatment

TSC offers a lifetime of treatment challenges for the various manifestations the disease including seizure control, management of cognitive and behavioral effects, and treatment for and monitoring of SEGA. For asymptomatic tumors, surveillance with gadolinium-enhanced MRI every 1–3 year in children and yearly in adults is recommended [31]. Surgery is recommended for symptomatic tumors or asymptomatic tumors in which growth or

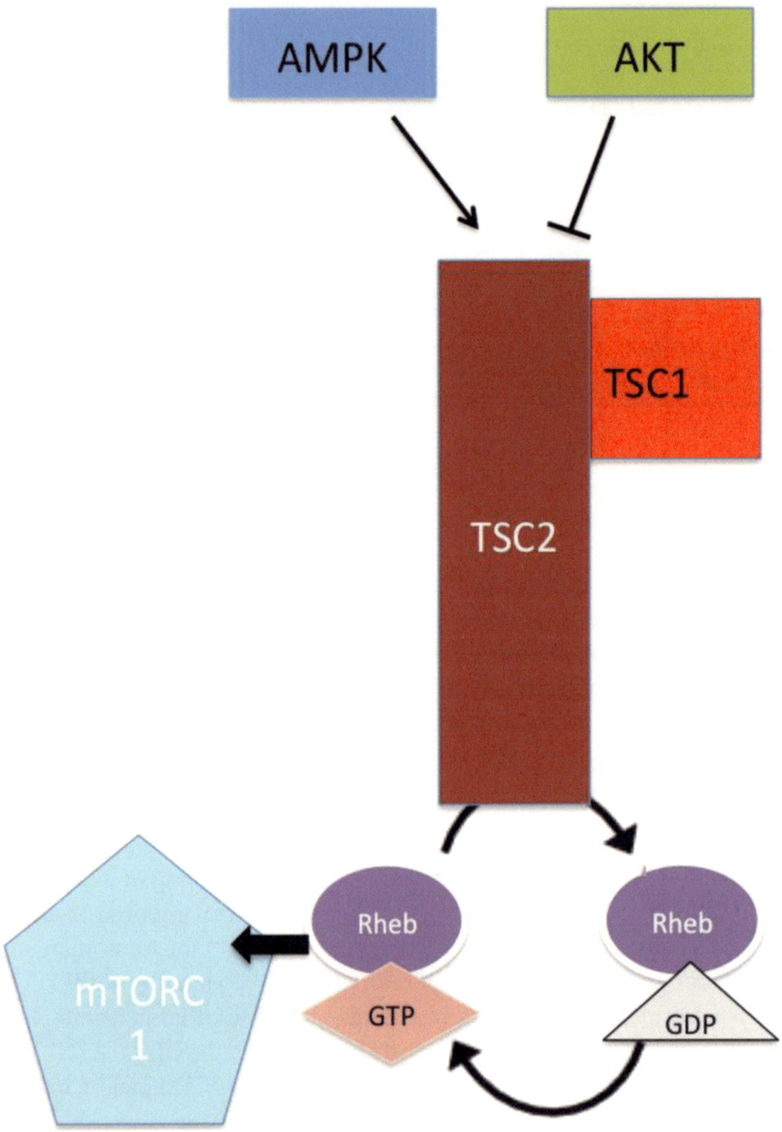

Figure 3. TSC 1 stabilizes TSC2 which is activated by AMPK and inhibited by AKT. The GAP domain of TSC2 inactivates mTORC1 by dephosphorylating GTP associated with Rheb (adapted with permission from Ref. [30]).

increase in ventricle size has occurred. Complete resection is curative, but incomplete resection may lead to tumor regrowth [32, 33], and ventriculoperitoneal shunting is often employed in addition to or in place of tumor resection in order to address the obstructive hydrocephalus resulting from SEGA growth at the foramen of Monro. Though radiation therapy has also been used to treat SEGA, it is not the standard of care and radiation-induced neoplasms have been reported [34].

Because TSC is caused by mutations in tumor suppressor genes leading to upregulation of the mTOR pathway, various mTOR inhibitors have been investigated as possible candidates to treat TSC. Inhibition of mTOR by rapamycin was shown to reduce the size of SEGA [35, 36], renal angiolipomas [37] lymphangioleiomyomatosis [38], and facial angiofibromas [39]. Everolimus [40], a derivative of rapamycin and an inhibitor of mTORC-1, was subsequently chosen as a possible therapy for patients with TSC. In a prospective, open-label Phase 2 study of 28 patients with SEGA, treatment with everolimus for 6 months resulted in reduction in tumor volume and seizure frequency was largely stable to improved [41]. This lead to a larger Phase 3 trial in which 117 adults with SEGA were randomized to receive either everolimus or placebo. Patients in the treatment group were found to have at least a 50% reduction in tumor volume versus the placebo group. Adverse effects were mostly mild and included seizures and stomatitis [35]. Consequently, in 2010, everolimus was FDA-approved for treatment of patients with SEGA that require therapeutic intervention but cannot be curatively resected.

2.5. Future directions

Treatment of TSC involves management of symptomatic SEGA, and recently, everolimus and rapamycin have offered a medical therapy to supplement surgery in treating these slow-growing but clinically important tumors. Currently, these agents are being investigated to manage other manifestations of TSC. Topical rapamycin is being studied to treat facial angiofibromas, and both rapamycin and everolimus are being investigated as treatment for renal angiomyolipoma. As the genetics of TSC are better understood, new molecular targets are likely to be discovered allowing novel pharmacologic agents the ability to improve the quality of life for patients afflicted with TSC.

3. Neurofibromatosis 1

3.1. Introduction

Neurofibromatosis Type 1 (NF1), also known as von Recklinghausen disease, is one of the most common autosomal dominant neurogenic disorders. NF1 affects about 1 in 3000 live births [42] and is sometimes referred as peripheral neurofibromatosis. Although the penetrance is autosomal dominant, there are about 50% sporadic mutations as well. The NF-1 gene is a tumor suppressor gene located on chromosome 17 (17q11.2) [43] and encodes the 250 kDa protein neurofibromas, which is involved in the regulation of the RAS family proto-oncogenes and in the mTOR pathway. The RAS pathway involves a complex downward complex pathway involved in cell differentiation and cell growth through GTP signaling. Mutations in the RAS gene can cause permanent cellular transduction consequently causing increased cellular proliferation causing tumor growth [44].

3.2. Diagnosis

The diagnostic criteria of neurofibromatosis include the presence of two or more of the following:

1. First degree relative with NF1.
2. Axillary of inguinal freckling.
3. Two or more neurofibromas or 1 plexiform neurofibroma.
4. Optic glioma.
5. Osseous lesions.
6. Two or more Lisch nodules.
7. Six or more café au lait spots measuring more than 5 mm in prepubertal individuals or more than 15 mm in postpubertal individuals number [45].

Genetic testing is of diagnostic importance but would not be able to predict the disease severity and outcome. Clinical manifestations of the disease include cutaneous manifestations such as cafe au lait spots, facial, and axillary freckling (Crowe's sign), generalized hyperpigmentation, juvenile xanthogranuloma, Lisch nodules (pigmented hamartomas of the iris), pseudoatrophic macules, and nevus anemicus (a congenital vascular anomaly that presents as a hypopigmented macule or patch). Glomus tumors, benign neoplasms arising from the glomus body of the dermis often occur under the nail or on the fingertips of patients with NF1, as does an increased incidence of melanoma. In addition, NF1 is associated with scoliosis, dysplasia of long bone (sphenoid wing dysplasia), macrocephaly, short stature, learning disabilities, and ADHD. Of course, the hallmark of NF1 is the presence of cutaneous and plexiform neurofibromas, benign (WHO Grade I) nerve sheath tumors arising from nonmyelinating Schwann cells which typically surround small diameter peripheral axons. In contrast, myelinating Schwann cells cover larger diameter peripheral axons and are not tumorigenic. Histologically, neurofibromas consist of elongated wavy cells with small dark oblong nuclei. The tumor is characterized by tortuous proliferation of all components of peripheral nerves including axons, Schwann cells, fibroblasts, and perineural cells. Plexiform neurofibromas are typically larger tumors with more extensive involvement and have the potential to transform into malignant peripheral nerve sheath tumors (MPNST), sarcomas that typically appear in adulthood. About half of MPSNT occur in patients with NF1 [46]. Optic Gliomas are benign tumors of the optic nerve, chiasm, or tract that affect 15–40% of children with NF1 [47]. They typically present with painless vision loss or proptosis and may demonstrate an afferent pupillary defect and optic nerve pallor.

3.3. Genetics

The NF1 gene encodes a large cytosolic protein called neurofibromin and has one of the highest rates of mutations in the human genome. It is about 60 exon and 300 KB of genomic DNA [48]. NF1 is an autosomal dominant disorder, but sporadic mutation occurs in about 50% of patients. The symptoms usually start around age 10 and the penetrance reaches 100% by age 20. NF1 is associated with many other cancers systemically including gliomas, pheochromocytoma, juvenile myelomonocytic leukemia as well as meningioma [49]. NF1 is expressed in neurons, oligodendrocytes, and Schwann cells, and acts as a tumor suppressor by negatively regulating signaling through the Ras pathway by virtue of its GTPase-activating protein (GAP) domain [50]. Over one thousand mutations have been identified in

NF1which lead to upregulation of the Ras signaling pathway leading to cell proliferation, migration, and differentiation.

3.4. Treatment

As per the guidelines from American Academy of Pediatrics children with NF1, routine MRI, EEG, and other imaging of the peripheral nervous system are no longer recommended. Instead they recommend getting routine neurological and ophthalmological examination unless specific other needs arises to image CNS and PNS. With the multitude of symptoms of neurofibromatosis 1, the treatment options available are limited. Surgery may be used to remove painful peripheral neurofibromas but is typically withheld for asymptomatic lesions. Resection is not possible for optic gliomas, though optic sheath fenestration is possible as is debulking of plexiform neurofibromas that involve the orbit.

Although radiation is used to control the local spread of these tumors in the CNS, they are side effects including emergence of other malignancies in the CNS, which limit their use [51]. Neurofibromas are generally considered to be chemoresistant but various chemotherapeutic agents have been investigated to treat MPNST including doxirubicin and ifosfamide but none have shown improvement in recurrence or survival.

3.5. Future directions

Although most of the management of NF1 is symptomatic, clinical trials are being performed to evaluate lovastatin [52] and lamotrigine [53], see whether these agents help with neurocognitive dysfunction. Rapamycin, an MTOR inhibitor, is being investigated as treatment for the plexiform neurofibromas but has not shown an effect on tumor size, though pain is improved with treatment [54, 55].

Imatinib, a tyrosine kinase inhibitor, shows promise in reducing the size of peripheral neurofibromas [56, 57]. Carboplatin and vincristine have also showed promise in treating low-grade gliomas in children with NF1 [58]. Topical vitamin D3 analogues had measurable clinical and histological effects for cutaneous lesions with notable lightening of the lesions and an increase in melanin incontinence.

4. Neurofibromatosis 2

4.1. Introduction

NF2 is also sometimes called central neurofibromatosis due to its predilection towards cranial nerve 8 and meningioma. It accounts for only 5–10% cases of all neurofibromas [59, 60], and there are few if any cutaneous findings. NF2 is an autosomal dominant disorder caused by the mutation in the merlin or schwannomin gene on chromosome 22 (q11–13.1). The precise mechanism as how this tumor suppressor gene manifests the disease is still not clear, but some of the studies have suggested gene activation signaling pathway in glioma tumor suppression [61]. The incidence of this disease is 1:25,000 [62], and it usually presents during adolescence with hearing loss and imbalance secondary to vestibular schwannoma. This disease is associated with the development of schwannoma, meningiomas, and other neural tumors. The disease course of the NF2 varies from individuals with mean age of onset of 22 years of age, and mean survival from diagnosis was 15 years and mean age of death at approximately 42 years of age [63]. The most common cause of mortality in NF2 is from rapid tumor growth causing increased intracranial pressure and compression of the brain stem. Morbidity is greatly increased with bilateral deafness and vestibular dysfunction. Usually, the earlier age of onset is associated with rapid growth in the tumor than a later age onset [64].

4.2. Diagnosis

The diagnostic criteria for NF2 (the Manchester criteria) requires one of the following:

1. bilateral Vestibular Schwannoma (VS)
2. one or more 1st degree relative with NF2 + unilateral vestibular schwannoma at <30 years
3. two of the following: multiple meningioma, glioma, schwannoma, juvenile posterior lenticular opacities

NF2 may present clinically with hearing loss or tinnitus or the sequelae of intracranial glioma or meningioma and schwannoma. Ophthalmological manifestations including juvenile posterior subcapsular cataracts, cortical wedge cataracts, retinal hamartomas, and epiretinal membranes. Cutaneous features are similar but less prominent than those in NF1.

Vestibular schwannoma are Grade I tumors, which histologically demonstrate uniformly spindled Schwann cells with Antonin A (cellular fascicular) and Antoni B (myxoid; vacuolated) regions. Nuclear pleomorphism, xanthomatous change, and vascular hyalinization are common, and Rosenthal fibers (bundles of clumped intermediate filament proteins) may be present.

4.3. Genetics

NF2 is an autosomal dominant disorder, although about 50% of the individuals were also found to have spontaneous mutations with no prior family history of NF2. Although the transmission risk is 50% in subsequent generations in parents who have NF2 and is <50% in isolated patients due to mosaics [65]. Tumor linkage analysis genetic testing is a great tool in patients who have sporadic mutation [66].

The NF2 gene product, merlin, is a scaffolding protein linking actin filaments to membrane glycoproteins, and its tumor suppression properties may be due to effects on contact-mediated growth inhibition, though the mechanism is currently poorly understood.

4.4. Treatment

The goal of management of patient with NF2 is to preserve quality of life. Genetic counseling is available to first-degree relatives of affected individuals. Regular MRI screening every 2 years for those high-risk individuals <20-year old and every 3–5 years for those age >20 years should be sufficient. In high-risk patient with positive family history, initial screening can be even started at age 10 years and they are after annual MRI should be sufficient [67]. Regular neurological examination is also of prime importance in these patients. Close surveillance is the key after successful surgery to look for any recurrences.

Surgery for vestibular schwannomas carries the risk of hearing loss [68] and possible injury to the facial nerve [69]. The typical treatment for vestibular schwannoma associated with neurofibromatosis is stereotactic radiosurgery with gamma knife [70]. This type of surgery is associated with better outcome in terms of hearing preservation in about of the patients. This is also associated with reduced recurrence of the tumor in one the study by decreasing the volume of tumor by 33%. [71, 72]. Although a number of complications have also been reported with surgical removal of the VS including air embolism, ICH, Ischemic stroke in the first 3 days of surgery. In one of the study, removal of contralateral VS was associated with increased growth of the other VS after surgery. Due to close proximity of the facial nerve, there are numerous facial nerve complications that can increase the morbidity in surgical patient [73]. Spinal meningiomas and schwannomas if producing neurological complications would need emergent surgery but in asymptomatic patients, they can be closely observed [67].

4.5. Future directions

The vascular endothelial growth factor (VEGF) inhibitors, PTC 299, and bevacizumab [74] have been studied for treatment of vestibular schwannomas in NF2 patients with some improvement in tumor size and hearing function. Lapatinib, which inhibits the tyrosine kinase associated with epidermal growth factor receptor and HER2/neu, has shown promise in adult and pediatric NF2 patients with progressive vestibular schwannomas. Newer gene therapy involving oncolytic recombinant herpes simplex vector has also been shown to reduce volume of the tumor. Curcumin, a HSP 90 inhibitor is also another potential pathway target but still in early part of development [75, 76].

5. Von Hippel–Lindau syndrome

5.1. Introduction

Von Hippel–Lindau (VHL) syndrome is an autosomal dominant disorder characterized by visceral cysts and benign tumors in multiple organ systems that have subsequent potential for malignant change. The disease is named after the German ophthalmologist Eugen von Hippel and the Swedish Pathologist Arvid Lindau. These tumors mainly include hemangioblastomas of CNS and retina (60–65%), renal cysts and carcinomas (40–45%). Tumors that occur less frequently include endolymphatic sac tumor, adrenal pheochromocytoma, epididymal, and broad ligament cystadenomas. A clinical classification system divides individuals who are affected by VHL disease into two groups: Those predominantly without pheochromocytoma are classified as VHL type 1, and those predominantly with pheochromocytoma classified as VHL type 2. VHL type 2 is further subdivided into type 2A (with renal cancer) and type 2B (without renal cancer). In type 2C, affected patients develop solely pheochromocytoma. The incidence of VHL disease in the United States is approximately 1 case in 36,000 live births. Males and females are affected equally, and it affects people of all ethnic groups. Age at diagnosis varies from infancy to age 60–70 years of age, with an average of 26 years [77].

5.2. Diagnosis

Von Hippel–Lindau (VHL) affects selective organs with the development of hemangioblastomas. This disease should be considered when hemangioblastomas is diagnosed before third decade, spinal cord is involved, and there are multiple other CNS or peripheral lesions. Melon and Rosen established diagnostic criteria for von Hippel–Lindau disease; for diagnosis, a patient must have at least 1 characteristic lesion in the central nervous system, eye, or viscera if there is a family history of an affected first-degree relative, or they must have 2 lesions in the absence of a family history [78]. Diagnosis is established by contrast enhanced MRI of the head and spine which characteristically identifies a solid-enhancing nodule associated with a pseudocyst or syrinx for CNS hemangioblastomas.

Signs and symptoms of hemangioblastomas are determined by tumor site, edema associated with it, cyst formation and spread. Absolute size and the rate of growth does not dictate the symptoms for tumors in all locations and the likely time for symptoms to appear for individual lesions remains unclear because of the saltatory growth pattern exhibited by many tumors [79]. A number of tumor types and organ systems are affected in VHL:

1. CNS hemangioblastomas are the main component of VHL disease that may occur either synchronously or metachronously. Roughly, 80% develop in the brain and 20% in the spinal cord. Growth patterns of these lesions can be saltatory (72%), linear (6%), or exponential (22%). Increased growth of CNS HGB was associated with male sex, younger age group, symptomatic tumors and hemangioblastoma-associated cysts. This indicates the role of biological features related to developmental processes, hormonal factors, other systemic factors, and/or proteasomal processing [79]. Recent studies show that pregnancy has no impact on CNS hemangioblastoma development or progression [80]. Within the brain, the majority are infratentorial, mostly in the cerebellar hemisphere. Supratentorial hemangioblastomas mostly develop in pituitary stalk. Headache, vomiting, and gait disturbances or ataxia is seen with infratentorial tumors; with tumors above the tentorium, symptoms depend on the location of the lesion.

2. Spinal tumors are mostly intradural, involving cervical or thoracic regions most frequently. Most symptom-producing spinal hemangioblastomas are associated with cysts/syringomyelia/syrinx [81]. They usually present with pain; cord compression may lead to sensory and motor loss.

3. Retinal hemangioblastomas, sometimes called retinal angiomas, are histologically identical to CNS hemangioblastomas. They may be the early manifestations of VHL syn-

http://dx.doi.org/10.5772/66207

drome and can occur in childhood with mean age of detection about 25 years. They are mostly located in the temporal periphery of the retina 90% or may develop in the posterior pole (1%) and optic disc (8%) [82]. Retinal hemangioblastomas may be asymptomatic or present with a visual field defect or a loss of visual activity due to retinal detachment, exudation, or hemorrhage. Retinal function tests are helpful in early detection of asymptomatic patients with quiescent retinal angiomas. The number of retinal angiomas does not appear to increase with age; however, there is greater likelihood of vision loss with age.

4. Renal manifestations of VHL include renal cysts or carcinomas. Renal cell carcinoma (RCC) is specifically of the clear cell subtype, which may develop either within a cyst or in the surrounding parenchyma. It occurs in 70% of affected individuals by sixth decade. RCC occurring in VHL is known to have similar growth kinetics as those of sporadic one [83]. A hallmark feature of clear cell renal cell carcinoma is that cells undergo a metabolic shift consistent with the Warburg effect. It is a leading cause of mortality in VHL syndrome, therefore, renal screening is very important [84].

5. Pancreatic cysts: Most pancreatic lesions in VHL are simple cysts that can be numerous in individuals with VHL. They rarely cause endocrine or exocrine insufficiency. Cysts in the head of the pancreas cause biliary obstruction.

6. Neuroendocrine tumors: 5–17% of individuals with VHL develop neuroendocrine tumors of the pancreas. They are not usually hormonally active and are slow growing. Malignant behavior has been observed in tumors >3 cm [85].

7. Pheochromocytoma: These may present with sustained or episodic hypertension or be totally asymptomatic, detected incidentally by an abdominal imaging procedure. Pheochromocytomas are usually located in one or both adrenal glands. They are usually benign, but malignant behavior has been reported.

8. Endolymphatic sac tumors: These are seen in approximately 10–16% of individuals with VHL syndrome, and in some instances, the associated uni- or bilateral hearing loss is the initial feature of the syndrome [86]. The onset of hearing loss is typically sudden; severity varies, but it is often severe to profound [87]. Vertigo or tinnitus is the presenting complaint.

Epididymal and broad ligament cystadenomas: Epididymal or papillary cystadenomas are relatively common in males with VHL syndrome. They rarely cause problems, unless bilateral, in which case they may result in infertility. The equivalent, much less common, lesion in women is a papillary cystadenoma of the broad ligament.

5.3. Genetics

VHL is caused by mutations of the VHL tumor suppressor gene on the short arm of chromosome 3 (3p25–26), and there are over 1500 known mutations to date. The VHL protein regulates the function of hypoxia inducible factor alpha (HIFα) by ubiquitinating it, leading to its degradation

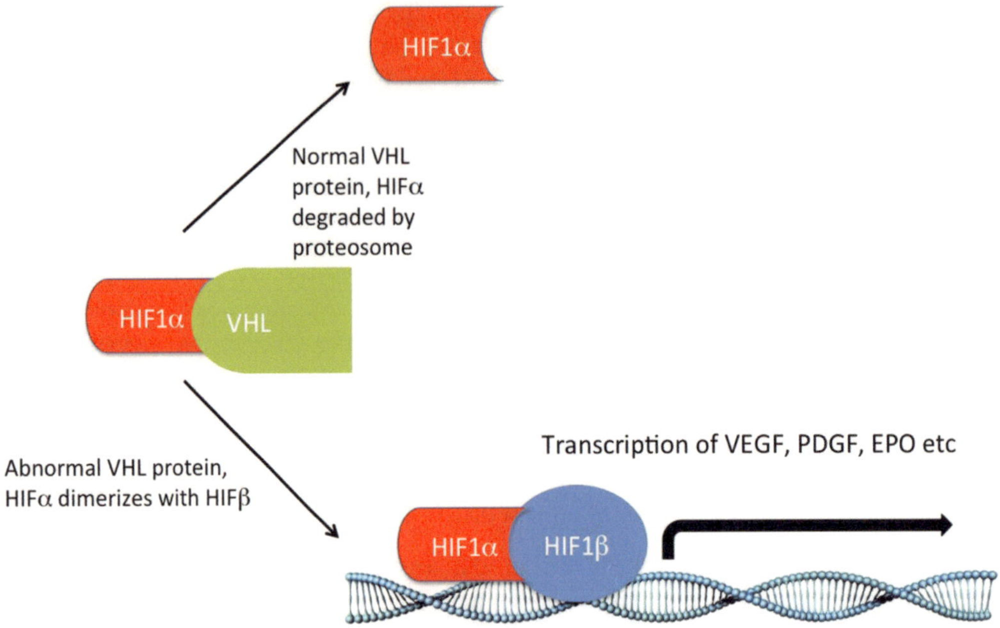

Figure 4. VHL binds to HIFα targeting it for proteosome degradation. With abnormal VHL protein, HIFα dimerizes with HIFβ and activates transcription of a number of genes involved in cell growth and differentiation (adapted with permission from Ref. [99]).

[88]. In VHL, HIFα is not degraded and instead dimerizes with HIFβ to activate the transcription of a number of genes including vascular endothelial growth factor, platelet-derived growth factor B, and erythropoietin [89] leading to multiple tumor types in various organ systems (**Figure 4**).

5.4. Treatment

CNS Hemangioblastomas: Surgery is the treatment of choice. The correct use of microsurgical techniques and thorough understanding of the anatomy yields satisfactory results with minimal morbidity and maximum functional recovery. Outcome depends upon the neurological status before surgery, site, and size of lesion [90]. Favorable results can be achieved by careful dissection of the tumor and preoperative embolization to prevent hemorrhage. The use of intraoperative ICG video angiography in recent years is very helpful for easily locating the minor feeding arteries and maintaining normal perfusion especially in spinal hemangioblastoma surgery [91]. Radiation may be considered if surgery is not suitable. Current medical therapy includes Bevacizumab, Vorinostat, and Dovitinib [92]. Extended periods of follow-up (5 years or more) are necessary to accurately assess the efficacy of nonsurgical therapies, such as chemotherapy and radiation therapy, and tumor stability. Current guidelines recommend that asymptomatic patients who present with a primary spinal cord tumor undergo observation. Symptomatic patients should undergo surgical resection as it promises acceptable rates of neurological improvements

Retinal hemangioblastomas: Most ophthalmologists favor prospective treatment of retinal (but not optic nerve) angiomas to avoid blindness. Laser photocoagulation is the treatment of choice for retinal capillary hemangiomas in the peripheral areas with a diameter of less than one-fourth of a disc. Cryotherapy is suitable for larger peripheral lesions. Vitrectomies may be useful for cases in which tractional retinal detachment has occurred. Despite being the mainstays of treatment, these procedures have their limitations; therefore, PDT (photodynamic therapy) and intravitreal anti-vascular endothelial growth factor (VEGF) are being considered as treatment options. PDT can be helpful in reducing macular edema associated with RCH (retinal capillary hemangioma); however, it has limitations especially for juxtapapillary tumors [93]. VEGF has been tried recently, but the outcomes are variable [94].

Renal Tumors: Patients with clear cell renal cell carcinoma have limited therapeutic options, as it is unresponsive to chemotherapy and is highly resistant to radiation. Surgery is the best option for renal cell carcinoma. Depending on the size and location of the tumor, nephron-sparing or partial nephrectomy may be possible without compromising survival. Renal transplantation has been successful in individuals in whom bilateral nephrectomy was necessary. Interleukin-2 (IL-2) therapy has proved to be effective in patients with metastatic RCC [95].

Pheochromocytomas: Surgical removal of the tumor has favorable outcome with few recurrences. Partial adrenalectomy is the treatment of choice in children and early screening is recommended [96].

Pancreatic cysts and neuroendocrine tumors: Pancreatic cysts do not require surgical removal; however, tumor needs surgical resection if there is a high risk of metastasis [97].

For VHL associated hemangioblastomas, yearly investigation for craniospinal hemangioblastoma by MRI and yearly screening and follow-up for retinal angiomas is recommended. Annual abdominal ultrasound with triennial CT imaging for abdominal masses is postulated. Annual audiometry is to be performed for possible endolymphatic sac tumor; detailed radiographic imaging of the skull base should be performed upon abnormality in auditory testing. Investigations for cystadenomas of the epididymis and broad ligament only are mandatory on indication. Annual investigation for pheochromocytoma is recommended [98].

5.5. Future directions

Extensive studies, assessing the efficacy of various drugs are in different phases of clinical trials. It includes the role of 17AAG (17-allylamino 17-demethoxygeldanamycin) on RCC and the effects of Sunitinib in VHL patients who are unresponsive to conventional treatment. EYE001 is an experimental drug that seems to have promising results for the treatment of retinal HBG and associated vision loss by decreasing VEGF production.

6. Conclusion

The phakomatoses constitute a complex group of neurocutaneous syndromes with cutaneous, ocular, and neural involvement. Mutations have been identified in a variety of genes affecting multiple aspects of cell cycle regulation including kinase signaling cascades such as mTOR and Ras as well as transcription factors. Due to the multitude of disease manifestations in multiple organ systems, treatment options are limited. A more complete understanding of the molecular mechanisms underlying these important disorders will lead to the identification of molecular targets for the development of new pharmacologic and biologic therapies.

Author details

Muhammad Taimur Malik, Mohammed Faraz Majeed and Scott G. Turner*

*Address all correspondence to: sgturner@geisinger.edu

Department of Neurology, Geisinger Medical Center, Danville, PA, USA

References

[1] Osborne JP, Fryer A, Webb D. Epidemiology of tuberous sclerosis. Ann N Y Acad Sci. 1991;615:125.

[2] Curatolo P, Bombardieri R, Jozwiak S. Tuberous sclerosis. Lancet. 2008;372(9639):657.

[3] van Slegtenhorst M et al. Identification of the tuberous sclerosis gene TSC1 on chromosome 9q34. Science. 1997;277:805–808.

[4] European Chromosome 16 Tuberous Sclerosis Consortium. Identification and characterization of the tuberous sclerosis gene on chromosome 16. Cell. 1993;75:1305–1315.

[5] Niida Y et al. Survey of somatic mutations in tuberous sclerosis complex (TSC) Hamartomas suggests different genetic mechanisms for pathogenesis of TSC lesions. AJHG. 2001;69(3):493–503.

[6] Curatolo P. Neurological manifestations of tuberous sclerosis complex. Childs Nerv Syst. 1996;12:15–21.

[7] deVries, PJ et al. Tuberous sclerosis associated neuropsychiatric disorders (TAND) and the TAND checklist. Pediatr Neurol. 2015;52:25–35.

[8] Rowley SA, O'Callaghan FJ, and Osborne JP. Ophthalmic manifestations of tuberous sclerosis: a population based study. Br J Ophthalmol. 2001;85:420–423.

[9] Rakowski SK, Winterkorn EB, Paul E, Steele DJ, Halpern EF, Thiele EA. Renal manifestations of tuberous sclerosis complex: inci- dence, prognosis, and predictive factors. Kidney Int. 2006;70:1777–1782.

[10] Martignoni G et al. Renal disease in adults with TSC2/PKD1 contiguous gene syndrome. Am J Surg Pathol. 2002;26(2):198–205.

[11] Pode D, Meretik S, Shapiro A, Caine M. Diagnosis and management of renal angiomyolipoma. Urology. 1995;25:461–467.

[12] Adler J, Greweldinger J, Litzky G. "Macro" aneurysm in renal angiomyolipoma: two cases, with therapeutic embolization in one patient. Urol Radiol. 1984;6:201–203.

[13] Harding CO, Pagon RA. Incidence of tuberous sclerosis in patients with cardiac rhabdomyoma. Am J Med Genet. 1990;37:443–446.

[14] Johnson SR et al. Review panel of the ERS LAM task force. European Respiratory Society guidelines for the diagnosis and management of lymphangioleiomyomatosis. Eur Respir J. 2010;35(1):14–26.

[15] Northrup H and the International Tuberous Sclerosis Complex Consensus Group. Tuberous sclerosis complex diagnostic criteria update: recommendations of the 2012 International Tuberous Sclerosis Complex Consensus Conference. Pediatr Neurol. 2013;49:243–254.

[16] Sarnat HB, Flores-Sarnat L. Embryology of the neural crest: its inductive role in the neurocutaneous syndromes. J Child Neurol. 2005;20(8):637–643.

[17] Mühlebner A, van Scheppingen J, Hulshof HM, Scholl T, Iyer AM, Anink JJ, et al. Novel histopathological patterns in cortical tubers of epilepsy surgery patients with tuberous sclerosis complex. PLoS One. 2016;11(6):e0157396. doi:10.1371/journal.pone.0157396

[18] Fukutani Y, Yasuda M, Saitoh C, Kyoya S, Kobayashi K, Miyazu K, Nakamura I. An autopsy case of tuberous sclerosis. Histological and immunohistochemical study. Histol Histopathol. 1992;7(4):709–714.

[19] Buccoliero AM, Franchi A, Castiglione F, Gheri CF, Mussa F, Giordano F, Genitori L, Taddei GL. Subependymal giant cell astrocytoma (SEGA): Is it an astrocytoma? Morphological, immunohistochemical and ultrastructural study. Neuropathology. 2009;29(1):25–30.

[20] Braffman BH, Bilaniuk LT, Naidich TP, et al. MR imaging of tuberous sclerosis: pathogenesis of this phakomatosis, use of gadopentetate dimeglumine, and literature review. Radiology. 1992;183:227–238.

[21] Vézina G. Neuroimaging of phakomatoses: overview and advances. Pediatr Radiol. 2015;45(Suppl 3):S433–S442.

[22] Manoukian SB and Kowal DJ. Comprehensive imaging manifestations of tuberous sclerosis. Am J Roentgenol. 2015;204:933–943.

[23] Inoki K, Li Y, Xu T, and Guan K-L. Rheb GTPase is a direct target of TSC2 GAP activity and regulates mTOR signaling. Genes Dev. 2003;17(15):1829–1834.

[24] Laplante, M and Sabatini DM. mTOR signaling at a glance. Cell Science. 2009;122:3589–3594.

[25] Chong-Kopera H, Inoki K, Li Y, Zhu T, Garcia-Gonzalo FR, Rosa JL, Guan KL. TSC1 stabilizes TSC2 by inhibiting the interaction between TSC2 and the HERC1 ubiquitin ligase. J Biol Chem. 2006;281(13):8313–8316.

[26] Huang J and Manning BD. A complex interplay between Akt, TSC2 and the two mTOR complexes. Biochem Soc Trans. 2009;37(Pt 1):217–222.

[27] Huang J and Manning BD. The TSC1–TSC2 complex: a molecular switchboard controlling cell growth. Biochem J. 2008;412(2):179–190.

[28] Inoki K, Zhu T, Guan KL. TSC2 mediates cellular energy response to control cell growth and survival. Cell. 2003;115(5):577–590.

[29] Jung CH, Ro S-H, Cao J, Otto NM and Kim DH. mTOR regulation of autophagy. FEBS Lett. 2010;584(7):1287–1295.

[30] Dibble CC, Elis W, Menon S, Qin W, Klekota J, Asara JM, Finan PM, Kwiatkowski DJ, Murphy LO, Manning BD. TBC1D7 is a third subunit of the TSC1-TSC2 complex upstream of mTORC1. Mol Cell. 2012;47(4):535–546.

[31] Hyman MH, Whittemore VH. National Institutes of Health consensus conference: tuberous sclerosis complex. Arch Neurol. 2000;57(5):662–665.

[32] Goh S, Butler W, Thiele EA. Subependymal giant cell tumors in tuberous sclerosis complex. Neurology. 2004;63(8):1457–1461.

[33] Cuccia V, Zuccaro G, Sosa F, Monges J, Lubienieky F, Taratuto AL. Subependymal giant cell astrocytoma in children with tuberous sclerosis. Childs Nerv Syst. 2003;19(4):232–243.

[34] Matsumura H, Takimoto H, Shimada N, Hirata M, Ohnishi T, Hayakawa T. Glioblastoma following radiotherapy in a patient with tuberous sclerosis. Neurol Med Chir (Tokyo). 1998;38(5):287–291.

[35] Franz DN, Leonard J, Tudor C, et al. Rapamycin causes regression of astrocy- tomas in tuberous sclerosis complex. Ann Neurol. 2006;59:490–498.

[36] Koenig MK, Butler IJ, Northrup H. Regression of subependymal giant cell astrocytoma with rapamycin in tuberous sclerosis complex. J Child Neurol. 2008;23:1238–1239.

[37] Wienecke R, Fackler I, Linsenmaier U, Mayer K, Licht T, Kretzler M. Antitumoral activity of rapamycin in renal angiomyoli- poma associated with tuberous sclerosis complex. Am J Kidney Dis. 2006;48(3):e27–e29.

[38] Morton JM, McLean C, Booth SS, Snell GI, Whitford HM. Regression of pulmo- nary lymphangioleiomyomatosis (PLAM)- associated retroperitoneal angiomyolipoma post-lung transplantation with rapamycin treatment. J Heart Lung Transplant 2008;27:462–465.

[39] Hofbauer GF et al. The mTOR inhibitor rapamycin significantly improves facial an- giofibroma lesions in a patient with tuberous sclerosis. Br J Dermatol. 2008;159:473–475.

[40] Easton JB, Houghton PJ. mTOR and cancer therapy. Oncogene. 2006;25:6436–6446.

[41] Krueger DA et al. Everolimus for subependymal giant-cell astrocytomas in tuberous sclerosis. N Engl J Med. 2010;363:1801–1811.

[42] Friedman JM. Epidemiology of neurofibromatosis type 1. Am J Med Genet. 1999;89(1):1–6.

[43] Shen MH. Molecular genetics of neurofibromatosis type 1. J Med Genet. 1996;33:2–17.

[44] Johnson MR. Inactivation of NF1 gene in human melanoma and neuroblastoma cell lines without impaired regulation of GTP.Ras. PNAS. 1993;90:5539–5543.

[45] DeBella K, Szudek J. Use of National institutes of Health criteria for diagnosis of neurofibromatosis 1 in children. Pediatrics. 2000;105:608–614.

[46] D'Agostino AN et al. Sarcomas of the peripheral nerves and somatic soft tissues associated with multiple neurofibromatosis (Von Recklinghausen's disease). Cancer. 1963;16:1015–1027.

[47] Listernick R, Charrow J, Greenwald MJ, Esterly NB. Optic gliomas in children with neurofibromatosis type 1. J Pediatr. 1989;5:788–792.

[48] Gutmann DA, Collins FS. Recent progress toward understanding the molecular biology of von Recklinghausen neurofibromatosis. Ann Neurol. 1992;31(5):555–561.

[49] Fahsold R et al. Minor lesion mutational spectrum of the entire NF1 gene does not explain its high mutability but points to a functional domain upstream of the GAP-related domain. Am J Hum Genet. 2000;66(3):790–818.

[50] Corral T, Jiménez M, Hernández-Muñoz I, Pérez de Castro I, Pellicer A.NF1 modulates the effects of Ras oncogenes: evidence of other NF1 function besides its GAP activity. J Cell Physiol. 2003;197(2):214–224.

[51] Packer RJ, Gutmann DH, Rubenstein D, et al. Plexiform neurofibromas in NF1. Neurology. 2002;58(10):1461–1470.

[52] Mainberger F, Jung NH, Zenker M, et al. Lovastatin improves impaired synaptic plasticity and phasic alertness in patients with neurofibromatosis type 1. BMC Neurol. 2013;13:131.

[53] Effect of Lamotrigine on Cognition in NF1 [internet]. 2016. Available from: https://clinicaltrials.gov/ct2/show/NCT02256124 [Accessed: 2016-08-30].

[54] Bhola P, Banerjee S, Mukherjee J, et al. Preclinical in vivo evaluation of rapamycin in human malignant peripheral nerve sheath explant xenograft. Int J Cancer. 2010;126(2):563–571.

[55] Hua C, Zehou O, Ducassou S, Minard-Colin V, Hamel-Teillac D, Wolkenstein P, Valeyrie-Allanore L. Sirolimus improves pain in NF1 patients with severe plexiform neurofibromas. Pediatrics. 2014;133(6):e1792–e1797.

[56] Demestre M, Herzberg J, Holtkamp N, et al. Imatinib mesylate (Glivec) inhibits Schwann cell viability and reduces the size of human plexiform neurofibroma in a xenograft model. J Neurooncol. 2010;98(1):11–19.

[57] Robertson KA, Nalepa G, Yang FC, et al. Imatinib mesylate for plexiform neurofibromas in patients with neurofibromatosis type 1: a phase 2 trial. Lancet Oncol. 2012;13(12):1218–1224.

[58] Packer RJ, Ater J, Allen J, Phillips P, Geyer R, Nicholson HS, Jakacki R, Kurczynski E, Needle M, Finlay J, Reaman G, Boyett JM. Carboplatin and vincristine chemotherapy for children with newly diagnosed progressive low-grade gliomas. J Neurosurg. 1997;86(5):747–754.

[59] Evans DR. Neurofibromatosis type 2 (NF2): A clinical and molecular review. Orphanet J Rare Dis. 2009;4:16.

[60] Viskochil, D. Neurofibromatosis: A Handbook for Patients, Families, and Healthcare Professionals. Am J Hum Genet. 2005. 77: 681.

[61] Yau YK, Murray LB, Houshmandi SS, Xu Y, Gutmann DH, Yu Q. Merlin is a potent inhibitor of glioma growth. Cancer Res. 2008;68(14):5733–5742.

[62] Martuza RL, Ojemann RG. Bilateral acoustic neuromas: clinical aspects, pathogenesis and treatment. Neurosurgery. 1982;10(1):1–12.

[63] Evans DG, Huson SM, Donnai D, et al. A genetic study of type 2 neurofibromatosis. II. Guidelines for genetic counseling. J Med Genet. 1992;29(12):847–852.

[64] Kanter WR, Eldridge R. Maternal effect in central neurofibromatosis. Lancet. 1978;2 (8095):903.

[65] Selvanathan SK, Shenton A, Ferner R, et al. Further genotype-phenotype correlations in neurofibromatosis 2. Clin Genet. 2010;77(2):163–170.

[66] Evans DG, Bourn D, Wallace A, Ramsden RT, Mitchell JD, and Strachan T. Diagnostic issues in a family with late onset type 2 neurofibromatosis. J Med Genet. 1995;32(6):470–474.

[67] Gutmann DH, Aylsworth A, Carey JC, et al. The diagnostic evaluation and multidisciplinary management of neurofibromatosis 1 and neurofibromatosis 2. JAMA. 1997;278(1):51–57.

[68] Temple RH, Axon PR, Ramsden RT, Keles N, Deger K, Yucel E. Auditory rehabilitation in neurofibromatosis type 2: a case for cochlear implantation. Acta Otolaryngol. 2009;129(9):971–975.

[69] Evans DG, Huson SM, Donnai D, et al. A genetic study of type 2 neurofibromatosis in the United Kingdom. I. Prevalence, mutation rate, fitness and confirmation of maternal transmission effect on severity. J Med Genet. 1992;29(12):841–846.

[70] Hasegawa T, Kida Y, Kobayashi T, Yoshimoto M, Mori Y, Yoshida J. Long-term outcomes in patients with vestibular schwannomas treated using gamma knife surgery: 10 year follow up. J Neurosurg. 2005;102(1):10–16.

[71] Phi JH, Kim DG, Chung HT, Lee J, Paek SH, Jung HW. Radiosurgical treatment of vestibular schwannomas in patients with neurofibromatosis type 2: tumor control and hearing preservation. Cancer. 2009;115(2):390–398.

[72] Sharma MS, Singh R, Kale SS, Agrawal D, Sharma BS, Mahapatra AK. Tumor control and hearing preservation after Gamma Knife radiosurgery for vestibular schwannoma in neurofibromatosis type 2. J Neurooncol. 2010;98(2):265–270.

[73] Acoustic Neuroma. NIH Consensus Statement Online. 1991.9(4):1–24.

[74] Wong HK, Lahenranta J, Kamoun WS, et al. Anti-vascular endothelial growth factor therapies as a novel therapeutic approach to treating neurofibromatosis-related tumors. Cancer Res. 2010;70(9):3483–3493.

[75] Angelo LS, Wu JY, Meng F, et al. Combining curcumin (diferuloylmethane) and heat shock protein inhibition for neurofibromatosis 2 treatment: analysis of response and resistance pathways. Mol Cancer Ther. 2011;10(11):2094–2103.

[76] Tanaka K, Eskin A, Chareyre F, et al. Therapeutic potential of HSP90 inhibition for neurofibromatosis type 2. Clin Cancer Res. 2013;19(14):3856–3870.

[77] Kim JJ, Rini BI, Hansel DE. Von Hippel Lindau syndrome. Adv Exp Med Biol. 2010;685:228–249.

[78] Melmon KL., Rosen SW. Lindau's disease: review of the literature and study of a large kindred. Am J Med. 1964;36:595–617.

[79] Lonser RR et al. Prospective natural history study of central nervous system hemangioblastomas in von Hippel-Lindau disease. J Neurosurg. 2014;120(5):1055–1062.

[80] Ye DY et al. Effect of pregnancy on hemangioblastoma development and progression in von Hippel-Lindau disease. J Neurosurg. 2012;117(5):818–824.

[81] Wanebo JE, Lonser RR, Glenn GM, Oldfield EH. The natural history of hemangioblastomas of the central nervous system in patients with von Hippel-Lindau disease. J Neurosurg. 2003;98:82–94.

[82] Maher ER et al. von Hippel-Lindau disease: a clinical and scientific review. Eur J Hum Genet. 2011;19(6):617–623.

[83] Bausch B et al. Renal cancer in von Hippel-Lindau disease and related syndromes. Nat Rev Nephrol. 2013;9(9):529–538.

[84] Asserraji M and El Kharras A. From headache to kidney tumor; an example of von Hippel- Lindau disease. J Renal Inj Prev. 2015;4(3):104–106.

[85] Corcos O, Couvelard A, Giraud S, Vullierme MP, O'Toole D, Rebours V, et al Endocrine pancreatic tumors in von Hippel-Lindau disease: clinical, histological, and genetic features. Pancreas. 2008;37:85–93.

[86] Binderup ML, Bisgaard ML, Harbud V, Møller HU, Gimsing S, Friis-Hansen L, Hansen Tv, Bagi P, Knigge U, Kosteljanetz M, Bøgeskov L, Thomsen C, Gerdes AM, Ousager LB, Sunde L; Danish vHL Coordination Group. Von Hippel-Lindau disease (vHL). National clinical guideline for diagnosis and surveillance in Denmark. 3rd edition. Dan Med J. 2013;60(12):B4763.

[87] Choo D, Shotland L, Mastroianni M, Glenn G, van Waes C, Linehan WM, Oldfield EH. Endolymphatic sac tumors in von Hippel-Lindau disease. J Neurosurg. 2004;100(3):480–487.

[88] Kaelin WG. Von Hippel-Lindau disease. Ann Rev Pathol. 2007;2:145–173.

[89] Bader HL, Hsu T. Systemic VHL gene functions and the VHL disease. FEBS Letters. 2012;586(11):1562–1569.

[90] Joaquim AF et al. Intramedullary hemangioblastomas: surgical results in 16 patients. Neurosurg Focus. 2015;39(2):E18.

[91] Takeshima Y et al. Visualization of vascular structure of spinal hemangioblastoma using intraoperative indocyanine green videoangiography and temporary feeder occlusion. Eur Spine J. 2015;24(Suppl 4):S585–S589.

[92] Kim BY, Jonasch E, and McCutcheon IE. Pazopanib therapy for cerebellar hemangioblastomas in von Hippel-Lindau disease: case report. Target Oncol. 2012;7(2):145–149.

[93] Papastefanou VP et al. Photodynamic therapy for retinal capillary hemangioma. Eye. 2013;27:438–442.

[94] Baba T et al. Subretinal hemorrhage after photodynamic therapy for juxtapapillary retinal capillary hemangioma. Case Rep Ophthalmol. 2011;2(1):134–139.

[95] Coventry BJ and Ashdown ML. The 20th anniversary of interleukin-2 therapy: bimodal role explaining longstanding random induction of complete clinical responses. Cancer Manag Res. 2012;4:215–221.

[96] Aufforth RD et al. Pheochromocytoma Screening Initiation and Frequency in von Hippel-Lindau Syndrome. J Clin Endocrinol Metab. 2015;100(12):4498–4504.

[97] Keutgen XM et al. Evaluation and management of pancreatic lesions in patients with von Hippel-Lindau disease. Nat Rev Clin Oncol. 2016;13:537–549.

[98] Bamps S et al. What the neurosurgeon should know about hemangioblastoma, both sporadic and in Von Hippel-Lindau disease: A literature review. Surg Neurol Int. 2013;4:145.

[99] Pavlovich CP and Schmidt LS. Searching for the hereditary causes of renal-cell carcinoma. Nat Rev. 2004; 4:381–393

Section 6

Management of Primary and Secondary CNS Malignancies

Chapter 6

Current Management of Brain Metastases: Overview and Teaching Cases

Karolyn Au, Ying Meng, Suganth Suppiah,
Anick Nater, Rakesh Jalali and Gelareh Zadeh

Additional information is available at the end of the chapter

http://dx.doi.org/10.5772/66310

Abstract

Over the past two decades, increased global incidence of malignancy, improved systemic disease treatment with prolonged survival, and increased central nervous system (CNS) surveillance in cancer patients have all contributed to a rise in cerebral metastatic disease. As many patients retain good neurologic function, the approach to their management has shifted markedly; a pre-terminal prognosis and palliative treatment have been replaced by individualized care plans to prolong functional survival. However, the rapid shifts in disease characteristics, treatment options and emerging evidence can be challenging to navigate, and a rational approach to brain metastases is needed. We discuss the changing epidemiology of brain metastases and consider approaches to prognostic classification. We review current treatment modalities and discuss the significant studies pertaining to each, with emphasis on Level 1 evidence when available and cooperative group trials, as well as studies on adverse effects. To integrate the information presented, we offer case scenarios that highlight pertinent decision-making factors. The shift in care goal for cerebral metastases from symptom palliation to prolongation of survival is not only feasible, but in many cases indicated. The appropriate application of various treatment modalities must be considered in the context of individual patients and their primary cancer.

Keywords: brain metastases, surgery, whole-brain radiation, stereotactic radiosurgery, targeted therapy

1. Introduction

Brain metastases are the most frequent intracranial neoplasm in adults, and the most common intracranial metastatic site is the brain parenchyma [1–3]. Historically, intracranial dissemination represented a poor prognosis for cancer patients, best supportive care leading to an overall survival around 1–2 months [4]. Advances in systemic cancer management, however, as well as in local treatments for cerebral disease, have greatly altered the prognosis and survival for patients. Brain metastasis management is therefore an emerging area of interest in organ-specific metastasis research addressing standard protocols for local management, including rational use of surgical resection, stereotactic radiosurgery (SRS), adjuvant or exclusive whole-brain radiotherapy (WBRT), and emerging systemic therapies. As survival increases, considerations for maintenance of neurocognitive function and quality of life gain greater importance. Decision-making for treatment of brain metastasis patients should be carried out in a multi-disciplinary setting, incorporating expertise from surgeons, oncologists, radiation oncologists, psychologists, and rehabilitation therapists.

2. Epidemiology of brain metastases

A *single* brain metastasis refers to the presence of only one parenchymal lesion in the context of an active primary cancer and possible extracranial metastases. In contrast, *solitary* brain metastasis describes the presence of only one parenchymal deposit with controlled primary tumour and no other metastatic disease. A synchronous brain metastasis is one that is identified at the time of presentation of the primary cancer, while a precocious one presents prior to the primary malignancy.

The accurate global incidence of brain metastasis based on population study is unknown, with estimates ranging around 7–14 per 100,000 [5]. Among cancer patients, estimates of prevalence range from 8.5 to 9.6% [6, 7]. These numbers are likely low, as they come from relatively old studies in which imaging or histology were often incomplete or which ignored cerebral disease in seriously ill patients with symptomatic advanced cancer [1]. Autopsy series report higher rates; a 1963 series found CNS metastases in up to 24% of patients [8], and in 1978, Posner and Chernick found that 15% of patients with cancer had parenchymal brain dissemination [9].

The incidence of brain metastases appears to be rising, with several contributing factors [2, 10]. First, the global incidence of cancer is climbing, but mortality rates are declining as a result of improved detection and treatment [1, 11]. New chemotherapeutic agents have led to a better prognosis and longer survival for many cancers, but fail to prevent central nervous system (CNS) spread due to low penetration of the blood–brain barrier, thus allowing greater opportunity for development of intracranial disease [1]. For example, the agent trastuzumab, a targeted therapy for HER2-positive breast cancer with presumed low CNS penetrance, has altered the natural history of this disease and may have unmasked the CNS as a sanctuary site [1]. In addition, improvement in surveillance, particularly due to greater diligence in following patients who have cancer and integrating brain MRI imaging into these follow-ups (64% today *vs.* 14% 20 years ago), has revealed more cerebral lesions prior to symptom development. For instance, patients with a new diagnosis of small cell and non-small cell lung carcinoma (NSCLC) typically undergo routine screening brain MRI, and inclusion into many clinical trials requires negative screening brain MRI [2].

http://dx.doi.org/10.5772/66310

The incidence and prevalence of brain metastases is also influenced by patient-specific factors, such as race or site of primary tumour. African-Americans with lung, melanoma, or breast cancer, but not renal cancer, appear at greater risk of developing brain metastases than Caucasians [6, 12]. However, confounders such as variability in healthcare access and awareness may account for some racial differences.

Although any neoplasm can potentially disseminate to the brain, certain primary histologies exhibit a higher propensity to do so; a population-based study from the Metropolitan Detroit Cancer Surveillance System found that 19.9% of lung, 6.9% of melanoma, 5.1% of breast, 6.5% of renal, and 1.8% of colorectal cancers develop brain metastases [6]. The prevalence of the primary tumour also affects the incidence of cerebral disease; thus 39–56% of brain metastases arise from lung, 13–30% from breast, 6–11% from melanoma, 2–6% from renal, and 3–4% from colorectal cancers [13–15]. Of note, in 10% of cases, no primary cancer can be identified [3]. The histology of the primary tumour is a key determinant in almost all epidemiological aspects of brain metastasis, including incidence, time interval from diagnosis of primary tumour to occurrence of intracranial spread, prognosis, and survival. In addition, the influence of molecular and genetic features is being increasingly recognised. For instance, the occurrence of cerebral dissemination varies according to the molecular subtype of breast cancer: the incidence for patients with triple-negative tumours [human epidermal growth factor receptor-2 (HER2) non-overexpressed, and oestrogen and progesterone receptor (PR) non-expressed] is 25–46%; whereas, it is 7.6% for patients with luminal tumour A (HER2 non-overexpressed, oestrogen and progesterone receptors expressed, and low proliferation index) [3].

Although a specific gender susceptibility might exist, the primary tumour type is thought to play an important role in the fact that the incidence of brain metastasis is higher in women than men. The increasing incidence of lung cancer in women and the propensity of breast tumours to metastasise to the brain have contributed to reverse the trend of 20 years ago, when more males were diagnosed with brain metastases [6, 16].

The median age at diagnosis has remained fairly stable for the past 20 years, ranging from 57 to 63 years [1]. Primary cancer influences the age at diagnosis: lung cancer, 40–49 years; melanoma, renal, and colorectal cancer, 50–59 years; breast cancer, 20–39 years. The higher frequency of cerebral metastases in younger and/or African-American women with breast cancer could be explained by the larger number of triple-negative tumours in this population, a subtype associated with a high risk of CNS progression [1].

Brain metastasis remains associated with advanced cancer, and over the past 20 years the proportion of patients with intracranial spread who also harbour extracranial metastases has increased (44 *vs.* 14%). [17]. The number of patients presenting with only one brain metastasis has fallen from 63 to 29%, while the proportion of patients with three or more lesions has increased from 17 to 36%. In addition, detection of synchronous brain metastases, at diagnosis of primary tumour, is also more frequent (from 18 to 30%) [17]. These changes are likely due to the increased use of brain MRI imaging. At the same time, the median time interval from diagnosis of primary tumour to detection of cerebral metastasis has increased from 3 to 8 months, depending on the site of primary tumour: 2.6–7 months for lung cancer as opposed to 39–47 months for breast cancer [1].

The increase in concurrent extracranial metastases directly impacts the assessment of prognosis; the Radiation Therapy Oncology Group (RTOG) recursive partitioning analysis (RPA) classification correlates clinical factors with median survival [18]. The most favourable prognosis, with median survival of 7.1 months, is seen in Class 1 patients who have a Karnofsky performance score (KPS) of ≥70, age <65, and controlled primary tumour without extracranial metastases. Class 3 patients have KPS <70 and a median survival of 2.3 months and are considered poor prognosis. All other patients fall into Class 2, including those with KPS ≥70 but other unfavourable characteristics, such as uncontrolled primary tumour, extracranial metastases, or age ≥65; these have a median survival of 4.2 months. The past two decades have seen a shift in patients away from both the most favourable (19 to 7%) and most unfavourable (44 to 31%) classes to the intermediate class [17–19].

It is well-recognised that primary tumour type influences median survival, with ranges including 2.7–6.3 months for lung, 5.1–6 months for colorectal, and 4.8–10 months for melanoma. In addition, survival for breast cancer differs according to histological and molecular subtypes; median survival for inflammatory breast cancer is 2.9 months, triple-negative is 4.9 months, HER2 overexpressing receiving trastuzumab is 11.3–26.3 months, and hormone receptor-positive is 19–24 months [1]. The diagnosis-specific graded prognostic assessment (DS-GPA) further incorporates prognostic variables significant to particular primary tumours; for instance, while age, KPS, the presence of extracranial metastases and number of brain metastases are seen to influence survival in lung cancer, and age, KPS and receptor subtype affect breast cancer survival, only KPS and number of BM were significant factors in melanoma and renal cell cancer and only KPS in gastrointestinal cancer survival [20].

Accurate prognostic information is useful to optimise treatment for patients who may gain months to years of survival following intracranial progression and to avoid overtreating patients who will derive little benefit. A contemporary cohort of brain metastasis patients who received more local (surgical resection and stereotactic radiosurgery) and systemic (chemotherapy and targeted therapy) treatment compared with a historical cohort had minimal improvement in median survival (3.2 *vs.* 3.9 months). However, 1-year survival increased from 15 to 34%, increased survival was seen at all time points during follow-up, and some long-term survivors were observed [17]. Survival was dependent on presenting symptoms of brain metastasis and treatment received.

Improvements in local procedures, along with increasing availability of systemic therapies, have altered the prognosis for patients with brain metastases.

3. Overview of brain metastasis management

Brain metastasis is a devastating sequela of cancer and develops in 25–40% of that patient population [21–23]. It is associated with a high morbidity and mortality; without treatment, median survival after diagnosis is approximately 1 month [24]. Treatment options include whole-brain radiation therapy (WBRT), surgical resection, stereotactic radiosurgery (SRS), and systemic therapies. With maximal management the overall survival rate increases to 10–12 months, although some patients demonstrate a remarkable response to treatment [21, 23, 24]. As a result, there is an ongoing debate regarding the most effective treatment regimen.

Not all brain metastases are equal, and there are many factors to consider when deciding on an appropriate treatment plan. Brain metastases can be categorised as solitary, single, or multiple. Furthermore, patients can be classified by type of primary tumour, status of systemic disease, functional status, and age to determine their prognosis, using such systems as the Radiation Therapy Oncology Group (RTOG) recursive partitioning analysis (RPA), or diagnosis-specific graded prognostic assessment (DS-GPA). Evaluation of these factors is important in identifying patients who will likely benefit most from aggressive treatment, as well as avoiding overtreatment of patients who are unlikely to benefit. In patients with a favourable prognosis (RPA class 1, some class 2), increasing overall and functional neurological survival are reasonable goals and thus focal therapies form a major component of treatment, and outcome assessment includes neurocognition and quality of life. In patients with an unfavourable prognosis, management focuses on symptom palliation as needed.

3.1. Whole-brain radiation therapy

WBRT was historically the treatment of choice for brain metastases, given that it was noninvasive and provided symptom relief and a modest survival benefit to a group of patients with few options. In most centres presently, it is used for patients with an unfavourable prognosis due to their extracranial disease or high burden of brain metastasis, or poor functional status. It is also used as adjuvant to focal treatment modalities (surgery or SRS), in order to reduce local recurrence and development of distant metastases, as well as salvage therapy on intracranial recurrence.

Over 70% of patients diagnosed with brain metastasis have multiple brain lesions at the time of diagnosis [21, 23]. The primary goals of treatment are to palliate symptoms and maintain neurologic function, and in some cases to increase survival, by treating the existing lesions and decreasing the volume of micro-metastases. The RTOG showed that approximately 50% of patients experienced neurological improvement by 2 weeks after initiation of WBRT. Median survival was 15–18 weeks, and 21 weeks in patients who were ambulatory [25]. Surprisingly, the dosing regimen did not affect survival [25, 26]. The typical radiation schedule involves a 7–15-day course of whole-brain radiation with 1.5–4 Gy per fraction. In some circumstances, a single fraction of 6–8 Gy or a bi-weekly fractionation regimen may be appropriate, such as when multiple treatment sessions may be impractical for a debilitated patient or unfeasible due to resource constraints. Such protocols may result in both inferior control rates and increased neurocognitive adverse effects, so should be applied with caution. Not all tumour histologies respond equally to radiation therapy; small cell lung cancer, germ cell tumours and hematologic malignancies are highly radiosensitive, while renal cell carcinoma, melanoma, and sarcoma are relatively radioresistant.

Acute adverse effects of WBRT include hair loss, nausea, vomiting and increased cerebral oedema with worsening of neurological symptoms. Concerns about long-term neurocognitive effects have been raised over the past two decades, especially as survival for patients with metastatic cancer is increasingly prolonged. A 1989 retrospective review found that

1.9–5.1% of patients who underwent WBRT developed progressive dementia, ataxia, and urinary incontinence causing significant morbidity [27]. Although most patients who developed these complications were given 5–6 Gy per fraction, a dose much higher than what is usually given today, a decline in memory and learning function is recognised in patients treated with typical fractionation protocols for WBRT, detectable between 6 and 12 months after treatment and not reversible [28]. Yet patients with brain metastases have detectable neurocognitive decline even prior to any treatment, indicating that cognitive changes may be attributable to the presence of tumour [29] and that failure to control metastatic brain disease also has a significant adverse impact on neurocognitive function [30]. Recent studies have explored strategies to reduce the toxicity of treatment, such as hippocampal-avoidance WBRT, which uses intensity-modulated radiotherapy (IMRT) to reduce the radiation exposure of the hippocampal neural stem cell niche important to memory function. A phase II study found reduced decline in Hopkins Verbal Learning Test-Revised Total Recall (HVLT-R TR), with low progression of disease within the hippocampal avoidance area, compared with historical controls [31]. Other approaches include use of the NMDA receptor antagonist memantine during and following WBRT administration; a small randomised controlled trial of memantine *vs.* placebo did not show a difference in the primary endpoint of memory decline (as measured by HVLT-R Delayed Recall), but did demonstrate longer time to cognitive decline [32]. The effectiveness of neuroprotective strategies and indeed the optimal modalities for neurocognitive testing remain areas of study.

3.2. Surgery

Surgical resection is considered for patients with a single symptomatic lesion in an accessible location, with the goal of reducing mass effect (e.g. to improve neurologic deficit or reduce seizures), decreasing tumour burden, and obtaining a tissue diagnosis when brain metastasis is in the differential diagnosis.

Level 1 evidence provides support for effectiveness of surgery in single metastatic brain lesions in patients with good functional status and controlled systemic disease. Patchell et al. randomised 48 patients into 2 groups (surgery + WBRT *vs.* needle biopsy + WBRT) and found that overall survival was higher in the surgical group, with a mean survival of 40 weeks compared to 15 weeks ($p < 0.01$). There was also a lower incidence of recurrence in the surgical site and longer functional independence [33]. This was supported by the results of Vecht et al., who also found improved overall and functionally independent survival with surgery + WBRT *vs.* WBRT alone in patients with good functional status and controlled extracranial disease; when there was active extracranial disease, the median survival was 5 months regardless of treatment [34]. In contrast, Mintz et al. found no significant difference in survival between the surgical and non-surgical groups [35]. However, the patient population in this study had a higher percentage of active systemic disease and lower functional status, compared to the other studies; these randomised controlled trials together emphasise the influence of these prognostic factors.

The surgical treatment of multiple brain metastases is more controversial. These patients tend to have greater systemic disease burden and are generally expected to have a short survival, so aside from the occurrence of a large lesion or one causing significant mass effect, they

http://dx.doi.org/10.5772/66310

are regarded as poor candidates for surgical resection. A case-controlled study by Bindal et al. showed that the mean survival of patients who had all of 2 or 3 lesions resected was significantly longer than that of patients who underwent incomplete resection and was similar to that of patients who had a single metastasis that was resected [36]. However, this study did not control for the number and locations of lesions. In contrast, Paek et al. did not identify a difference in survival among patients who underwent resection of one versus two or three metastases [37]. Iwadate et al. found that total residual tumour quantity, rather than lesion number, was a significant predictive factor; an improvement in survival from 4.5 to 12.4 months was seen when patients with multiple brain metastases underwent a total or subtotal resection with cumulative residual tumour <2 cm ($p < 0.05$) [38]. Taken together, these observational studies and conflicting results do not support resection of multiple metastases for the purpose of tumour control.

Following surgical resection, local recurrence is common and adjuvant radiotherapy aims to eliminate tumour cells remaining within the tumour bed, as well as to reduce micro-metastases in other locations throughout the brain. However, while multiple retrospective series have shown that WBRT does decrease distant recurrence, it confers no survival benefit [39–41]. In a randomised controlled trial comparing surgery *vs.* surgery + WBRT for a single metastasis, adjuvant WBRT reduced the local recurrence rate from 46 to 10% ($p < 0.001$), distant recurrence from 37 to 14% ($p < 0.01$), and decreased the likelihood of death from neurological causes. Remarkably, WBRT reduced the rate of total intracranial progression from 70 to 18% ($p < 0.001$), but there was no overall survival benefit or difference in duration of functional independence [42]. The EORTC 22952 randomised controlled trial evaluated adjuvant WBRT *vs.* observation following local treatment, either surgical resection or radiosurgery. The probability of local and distant relapse was significantly reduced in the WBRT arm, after both surgery and SRS. Survival with functional independence (WHO performance status > 2) and overall survival did not differ between the two arms, and initial treatment (surgery or SRS) was not a significant factor [43].

Radiosurgery to the resection cavity following surgical excision has become increasingly utilised in order to spare the use of WBRT. Multiple retrospective series showed improved local control with the addition of adjuvant SRS to surgery, with rates comparable to adjuvant WBRT [44–46]. The first prospective study included 50 resection cavities, of which 40 received SRS and 10 were observed, and found a significantly lower rate of local failure in the SRS group (15 *vs.* 50%, $p = 0.008$) [47]. An ongoing phase III study through the Alliance for Clinical Trials in Oncology aims to provide level 1 evidence on this issue, randomising to WBRT or SRS patients with ≤4 metastases who have had ≥1 tumour resected. The primary endpoints will include overall survival and neurocognitive progression. As it stands, the high rate of local recurrence following surgery warrants adjuvant radiation, and the low morbidity of SRS to the tumour bed favours this combination of treatments to improve local control.

3.3. Stereotactic radiosurgery

In recent years, more patients are being managed with stereotactic radiosurgery, a non-invasive option for focal treatment of metastatic brain tumours. This technique was originally developed by Lars Leksell and utilises multiple convergent radiation beams on a tumour to deliver a highly focused and concentrated dose. It has the advantage of exhibiting a steep radiation dose drop-off outside the tumour border, thereby reducing radiation exposure to surrounding tissue. Metastatic brain tumours tend to be lesions with discrete borders and spherical shape, often less than 3 cm in size, making them ideal candidates for SRS. Its non-invasiveness allows SRS to treat lesions in surgically inaccessible locations, as well as multiple lesions in a single outpatient session. Additionally, its efficacy is similar among relatively radio-resistant histologies such as renal cell carcinoma and melanoma, compared to radiosensitive tumour types. A minimal marginal dose of 18 Gy is associated with improved local control [48], and dose prescriptions generally range 18–25 Gy, lower doses being favoured in the brainstem and other eloquent locations, and when combined with WBRT. It does not reduce mass effect, however, and toxicity and local failure increase with increasing tumour size. While the acute effects of SRS are generally well-tolerated, the most common delayed complication is radiation necrosis, which may occur in up to 10% of tumours, 6 months to several years after treatment. Radiation necrosis develops more frequently with higher radiation dose, following prior stereotactic or fractionated radiation treatment, in larger tumours, and possibly when SRS is combined with targeted or immune therapy [49]. Distinguishing treatment effect from tumour recurrence is necessary but challenging, as both can exhibit increased enhancement and peri-lesional oedema, and advanced imaging techniques such as perfusion MRI and amino acid PET are under investigation to increase diagnostic specificity. Treatment is largely symptomatic, with corticosteroids. Observational studies have explored treatment for severe cases including resection, laser interstitial thermal therapy, bevacizumab, or hyperbaric oxygenation [50].

The efficacy of SRS was demonstrated in a randomised controlled trial carried out by Kondziolka et al., which compared WBRT plus a single-dose radiosurgery boost to WBRT alone in patients with 2–4 brain metastases. At a planned interim analysis, the primary endpoint of local control so strongly favoured combination treatment that the study was stopped ($p = 0.0016$). This left it underpowered to demonstrate a difference in overall survival. At one-year follow-up, the rate of local failure was 100% in patients treated only with WBRT, compared to 18% in those who had received SRS boost ($p = 0.002$) [51]. The subsequent RTOG 9508 randomised controlled trial also comparing WBRT plus SRS to WBRT alone in patients with 1–3 tumours found that the primary endpoint of median survival was met in the combined treatment arm, but only in patients with a single lesion (6.5 *vs.* 4.9 months, $p = 0.04$). The secondary endpoints of local control and improvement in performance status were met in the whole treatment cohort [52]. A secondary analysis of this data by Sperduto et al. that stratified patients by GPA found that WBRT + SRS conferred a survival benefit in good-prognosis patients (GPA 3.5-4) even with >1 lesion [53]. As with surgery, these studies emphasise the significant prognostic effect of good pre-treatment function and controlled systemic disease.

In comparing stereotactic radiosurgery with surgical resection, multiple retrospective studies have shown comparable survival, with some suggesting improved local control for SRS [54, 55], others favouring surgery [56], and still others suggesting a similar local control rate for the two modalities [57]. A single randomised controlled trial comparing surgery + WBRT with SRS was stopped prematurely due to poor accrual; the data acquired showed similar rates of local recurrence, overall survival and neurological death between the two arms [58]. Overall, the data suggest that SRS is at least as effective as surgery for tumour control and given the collective experience with its safety and utility, in the absence of a specific surgical indication such as a large or symptomatic lesion or uncertain diagnosis, is appropriate as first-line treatment for 1–3 newly diagnosed brain metastases.

The use of adjuvant WBRT for SRS has been controversial, and several randomised controlled trials have compared SRS with adjuvant WBRT to SRS alone. Similarly to the EORTC 22952 results, the Japanese Radiation Oncology Study Group found no significant difference in the primary endpoint of overall survival, or in functional preservation, despite significant reduction in local and distant recurrence in the WBRT arm [59]. In a single-institution RCT, Chang et al. evaluated a primary endpoint of cognitive function as determined by HVLT-R TR. A planned interim analysis at 4 months found a higher rate of total recall deterioration in the SRS + WBRT arm, and the trial was therefore halted. At study conclusion, overall intracranial recurrence was reduced in the WBRT arm, but a survival benefit was seen in the SRS-alone arm, a difference from other studies that the authors attributed to salvage therapies [60]. A cognitive primary endpoint was evaluated in the multi-institutional study of Brown et al., deterioration defined as decline of >1 standard deviation on ≥1 of 7 instruments assessing a range of cognitive domains. Cognitive deterioration was significantly worse in the WBRT arm, as were quality of life measures. Intracranial relapse was significantly greater in the observation arm, but overall survival was not different [61]. The evidence supports consideration of close observation for intracranial progression following SRS for 1–3 metastases, with salvage therapy at that time, to avoid routine use of adjuvant WBRT.

Earlier series limited the use of SRS to ≤4 lesions, a restriction that was largely technical rather than biological, and currently multiple lesions can be easily treated in a single session. Yet the evidence that guides treatment of a few lesions cannot necessarily be extrapolated to the management of many tumours; for instance, although SRS is highly conformal, with increasing tumour number the intervening brain is exposed to more radiation. In addition, some series suggest that the number of tumours is less important than the total tumour volume. A prospective observational study in patients with 1 to 10 brain metastases treated with SRS found that patients with a single lesion experienced significantly longer survival, but showed no difference in survival between patients with 2–4 and 5–10 tumours [62]. These latter groups also showed no difference in local or distant failure, suggesting that up-front use of SRS may be as appropriate for ≥5 lesions as for ≤4. An ongoing trial through the North American Gamma Knife Consortium aims to shed light on the neurocognitive outcome of patients with multiple metastases randomised to either SRS or WBRT. Included are patients harbouring ≥5 lesions, with no maximum number but total tumour volume restricted to 15 mL. This study will additionally evaluate patient- and caregiver-assessed quality of life, and include a cost analysis.

At the time of intracranial progression, repeat SRS may be considered in patients who maintain a good functional status and controlled systemic disease. Imaging suggestion of local recurrence must be distinguished from treatment effect, and especially if minimally symptomatic, a conservative approach with serial imaging is generally warranted before repeat treatment. Risk factors for local recurrence may include larger tumours, lower marginal dose, and melanoma histology. Multiple retrospective series have shown efficacy for SRS in new or recurrent tumours, including after WBRT, with adjustment to lower fraction dose in the setting of prior radiation exposure. These series suggest a local control rate comparable to first-time SRS [63–65].

3.4. Systemic therapy

The use of cytotoxic chemotherapy in treatment of brain metastases has historically been limited due to the perception that the blood–brain barrier isolates tumour cells from circulation agents. Furthermore, these patients usually have already been heavily pre-treated with conventional chemotherapy for their primary cancer, this prior exposure leading to tumour resistance against many agents. In addition, death from progression of systemic disease may preclude an assessment of the effect of the agent on intracranial disease. However, some phase II clinical trials have shown promising results for newer drugs in the treatment of certain subtypes of metastatic brain lesions [66]. The DNA-alkylating agent temozolomide has been widely studied for the treatment of brain metastases, in large part due to its high blood–brain barrier penetrability. It has modest efficacy in monotherapy, but in combination with radiotherapy or other chemotherapeutic agents has demonstrated encouraging results, with up to 40% disease control in brain metastases from various primary sources as well as minimal drug-related toxicity [67–69].

A meta-analysis of platinum-based chemotherapeutic agents (e.g. cisplatin) for small cell lung cancer demonstrated a 66% response rate for patients with brain metastases at initial diagnosis and 36% response rate for delayed brain metastases [70]. Unfortunately, most patients suffered from relapse of their disease or toxic side effects such as febrile neutropenia and sepsis [71]. In non-small cell lung cancer (NSCLC), these agents have shown a 28–45% response rate in chemotherapy-naïve patients [72]. Inhibitors of epidermal growth factor receptor (EGFR) have been approved for treatment of NSCLC due to the identification of frequent *EGFR* mutations in these tumours, and some retrospective series have demonstrated effect in brain metastases [73–76]. A phase II study of erlotinib in NSCLC patients with asymptomatic brain metastases showed a 58% complete or partial response rate, including in some tumours without *EGFR* mutation. The median progression-free survival was significantly longer in mutant *EGFR* tumours than in wild-type tumours (15.2 *vs.* 4.4 months, respectively; $p = 0.02$) [77]. Other NSCLC tumours bear an oncogenic *EMI4-ALK* translocation, and 30% of these patients develop brain metastases [78]. The ALK-targeted tyrosine kinase inhibitor (TKI) crizotinib has demonstrated CNS penetration and effect, although patients invariably relapse [79]. Second-generation inhibitors of ALK may exhibit greater activity and durability of effect [80]. Combination of targeted agents with radiotherapy may be synergistic and yield improved response and survival, at the cost of increased adverse effects [81].

Patients with intracranial breast cancer metastases have response rates of 43–59% to cyclophosamide with various combinations of 5-fluorouracil, methotrexate, and vincristine [72]. The molecular subtypes of breast cancer demonstrate different tendencies for brain dissemination, with triple-negative and HER2-positive tumours carrying the highest risk [82]. Routine treatment of the latter group of patients with HER2-directed therapy has markedly improved the overall prognosis, but a number of studies have shown an increase in brain metastases in patients treated with trastuzumab [83]. This effect may be secondary to increased survival of patients with this agent and low permeability of the antibody through the blood–brain barrier [71, 72]. There is increasing interest in the role of agents such as lapatinib, a dual EGFR- and HER2-specific TKI, which has shown modest intracranial anti-tumour activity in phase II trials [84, 85]. In addition, the phase II LANDSCAPE trial evaluating the combination of lapatinib and capecitabine, an inhibitor of DNA synthesis, demonstrated a 66% partial response and suggested that this systemic treatment may be an alternative to WBRT in HER2-positive patients [86]. Further randomised controlled trials are ongoing to explore the role for these and other systemic agents.

Cerebral metastases in melanoma historically carried a dismal prognosis. Cytotoxic chemotherapy is largely ineffective in management of metastatic melanoma, but new biologically active agents have dramatically altered the course of both intra- and extracranial disease for some patients. A phase II study of the anti-cytotoxic T-lymphocyte antigen 4 (CTLA-4) monoclonal antibody ipilimumab demonstrated a 24% tumour control rate in patients asymptomatic from brain metastases, and a 10% control rate in symptomatic patients on steroid therapy. The survival of patients with limited brain metastases on ipilimumab was similar to that of patients who did not have CNS disease [87]. In addition, occasional long-term responses have been observed with ipilimumab [88]. Dabrafenib, a small-molecule BRAF inhibitor, has shown efficacy in melanoma containing a *BRAF* mutation; in a phase II trial, among melanoma containing the *BRAF* V600E mutation, an intracranial response was demonstrated in 39% of patients who had not previously undergone treatment for brain metastasis, and in 31% of patients who had progressive brain metastases after local treatment [89]. Even with bulky disease, BRAF inhibitors can rapidly improve symptoms and control intracranial disease, although the response is generally short-lived. Investigations are ongoing into the optimal strategies for combining and incorporating these agents into management plans, as well as into other strategies.

4. Illustrative cases for evolving clinical considerations in brain metastases

Continued improvement in managing primary and systemic malignancy combined with greater sensitivity in detection of intracranial dissemination has increased the clinical burden of cerebral metastases. However, advances in therapy including refined surgical techniques and operative adjuncts, stereotactic radiation, and targeted systemic agents have shifted the goals of management from symptom palliation and modest survival increase to potentially long-term maintenance of neurologic function, cognitive independence, and quality of life. While progress is being made on many fronts, the array of treatment options also leads to many new areas of uncertainty. The cases below highlight some of the challenges currently faced by clinicians caring for patients with brain metastases.

Case 1: Whole-brain radiotherapy and neurotoxicity

A 47-year-old man develops headaches and clumsiness of his left arm. He has no significant medical history and is employed as an accountant. MRI of the brain demonstrates

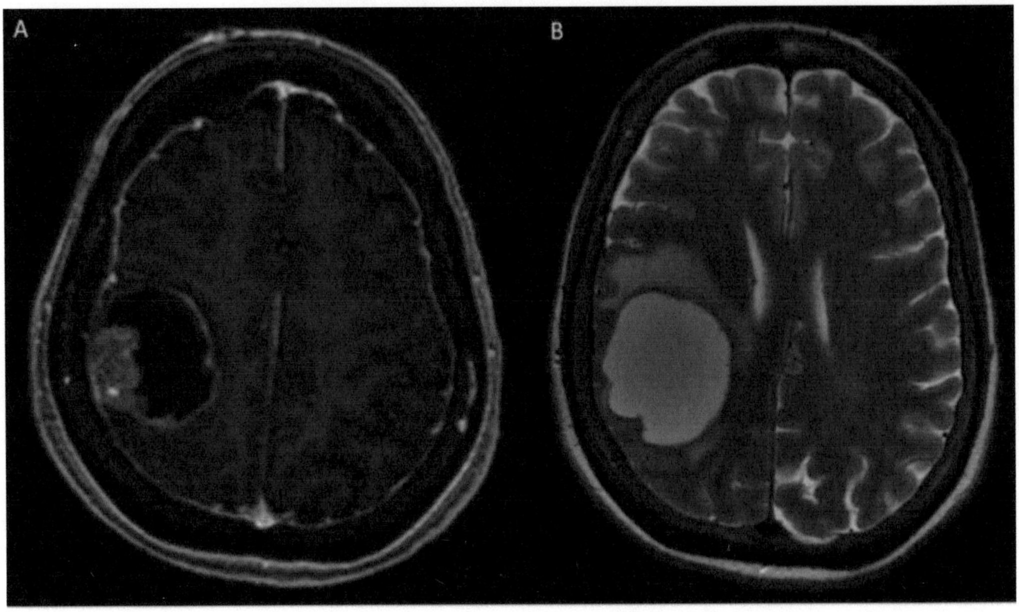

Figure 1. Pre-treatment (A) T1 with gadolinium contrast and (B) T2 MRI at initial presentation, showing a single large right-sided mass with oedema and mass effect.

a right frontoparietal enhancing 3 cm mass with associated cyst, with surrounding vasogenic oedema (Figure 1A and B). CT scan of the body reveals a pulmonary nodule but no other lesions. Due to the neurologic symptoms, he undergoes craniotomy, and the intracerebral lesion is metastatic adenocarcinoma consistent with lung primary. He makes satisfactory recovery from surgery with improvement of neurologic function. He wishes to receive aggressive treatment for the brain metastasis but hopes to continue working as long as possible.

Randomised controlled trial data indicate that intracranial recurrence following surgical resection of a metastasis can be as high as 70%. This same study showed that adjuvant whole-brain radiotherapy (WBRT) following surgery improves local control and decreases distant intracranial recurrence as well as neurologic mortality. Overall survival is unchanged [42]. Adjuvant WBRT following surgery is therefore recommended as a standard of management. However, many patients and physicians are increasingly concerned about the neurocognitive sequelae of WBRT, and some may wish to defer adjuvant WBRT in a patient with favourable prognostic factors (e.g. oligo-metastatic brain disease, good functional status, limited systemic disease) [27]. Retrospective studies report local control rates for SRS given to the tumour bed of a resected lesion that are comparable to post-operative WBRT [45, 46]. Patients must be counselled that intracranial progression also carries risk of neurocognitive deterioration.

In this case, SRS to the resection cavity would improve the rate of local control while sparing the neurocognitive adverse effects of whole-brain radiation. This patient requires close monitoring for the development particularly of new intracranial lesions.

http://dx.doi.org/10.5772/66310

Case 2: Local treatment of multiple metastases

A 52-year-old man presents with a 2-week history of word-finding difficulties and right leg weakness. He has a history of non-small cell lung cancer (NSCLC), negative for driver mutations, stage II at diagnosis, and treated 2 years prior. Four months ago, he received treatment for a single pulmonary metastasis, and on cytotoxic chemotherapy has demonstrated no recurrence. At this time, MRI of the brain shows two enhancing masses, a 3-cm medial left frontal lesion and a 3.5-cm left temporal tumour. The lesions are associated with extensive vasogenic oedema, and early uncal herniation is visible (Figure 2A and B).

Stereotactic radiosurgery is an acceptable first-line treatment for a limited number of cerebral metastases in patients with good function and controlled systemic disease. However, SRS does not reduce mass effect and may transiently worsen oedema, leading to increased neurologic deficits.

Symptomatic mass effect is rapidly and effectively decreased with surgical tumour excision, but patients with multiple cerebral metastases are generally expected to have a short survival, so are considered poor candidates for surgery. Only retrospective series are available to address the issue, and the data are unclear as to whether the number of lesions or the total volume has a greater impact on outcome. Nevertheless, consideration of surgery may be made

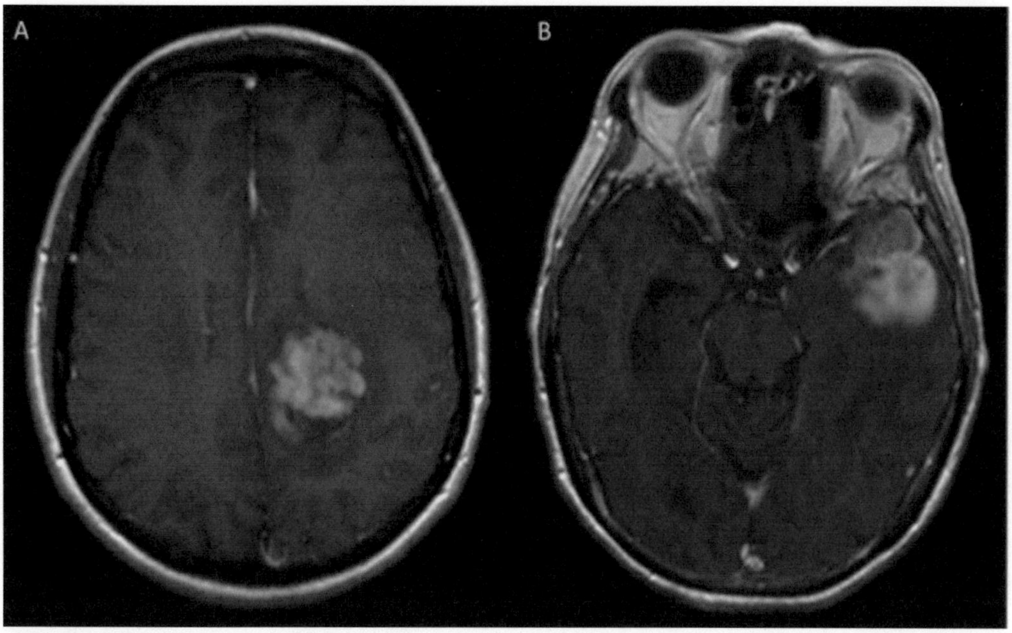

Figure 2. (A) and (B) Presenting T1 gadolinium contrast-enhanced MRI showing large left frontal and temporal lesions with oedema and mass effect.

for a large, symptomatic lesion among multiple, or for a lesion in a high-risk location for mass effect such as the cerebellum or temporal lobe.

Treatment decisions must consider the whole patient and consider the systemic context of their disease. At times, a decision is made on a case-by-case basis with discussion between the multidisciplinary management team and the patient. In this case, whole-brain radiation may be favoured, although surgical resection of the symptomatic lesion may be considered for rapid relief of mass effect.

Case 3: WBRT: alone, adjuvant or not at all

A 63-year-old woman presents to the emergency department with new-onset generalised seizure. She had a neck melanoma treated with local excision 2 years prior. Antiepileptic medication controls the seizures, and she has a normal neurologic exam. MRI of the brain demonstrates four enhancing cerebral lesions as well as two cerebellar lesions (Figure 3A and B). CT and PET scan of the body demonstrate no other lesions.

WBRT has traditionally been the mainstay of treatment for multiple cerebral metastases, as it provided a modest survival benefit to patients with a poor prognosis and few options [25]. However, improved treatment of primary and metastatic malignancy has altered the prognosis for many patients, and better strategies to control intracranial progression as well as reduce the neurotoxicity of WBRT have been sought. This is particularly true for metastatic melanoma, a disease with very poor prognosis that is also relatively radio-resistant. In patients with a limited number of brain metastases (≤4), randomised controlled trials

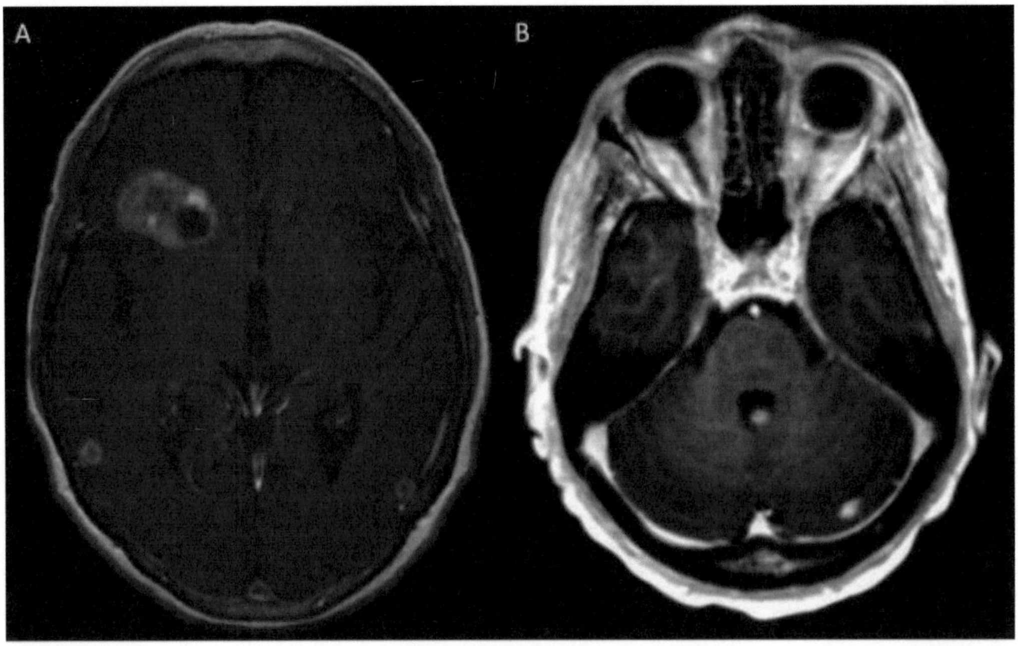

Figure 3. (A) and (B) Presenting T1 with gadolinium contrast MRI showing multiple enhancing cerebral lesions.

have demonstrated that addition of an SRS boost to WBRT improves local control compared to WBRT alone [51, 52]. More recently, a prospective series showed that multiple (2–10) tumours can be controlled with SRS alone, with no greater local or distant recurrence in patients with 5–10 lesions compared to 2–4 lesions [62]. Several randomised controlled trials have also shown that adjuvant WBRT following SRS compared to SRS alone decreases the rate of intracranial relapse at local and distant sites, although overall survival is not affected [90].

For some histologies, systemic treatment may be considered as an upfront treatment or as adjuvant to a local modality. In a phase II study, ipilimumab immunotherapy demonstrated effect against metastatic melanoma with intracranial involvement [87]. A retrospective study showed no difference in survival among patients with metastatic melanoma with or without intracranial involvement when treated with systemic ipilimumab [88]. Randomised controlled trial data are not yet available to directly compare the efficacy of WBRT with systemic therapies.

In this case, WBRT remains an acceptable treatment, although first-line SRS with close imaging follow-up may also be considered. Where available, immunotherapy may be offered.

Case 4: Radiation necrosis detection and management

A 56-year-old woman is referred for management of intracranial metastases identified on surveillance imaging (Figure 4A). She had HER2-positive breast cancer treated with mastectomy, and has been on trastuzumab therapy for 10 months with satisfactory control of primary disease and no evidence of systemic metastasis. MRI of the brain shows two small lesions, and she receives SRS (21 Gy to each of the two lesions in a single fraction) and a course of WBRT (20 Gy in 10 fractions). Follow-up imaging demonstrates that the lesions have decreased in size, and no new lesions have developed (Figure 4B). Ten months after treatment, the patient begins experiencing morning headaches. On MRI, the lesions have expanded in size with more avid enhancement and are associated with increased oedema (Figure 4C and D).

Radiographic progression of lesions treated with SRS may be evidence of tumour progression or of treatment effect (i.e. radiation necrosis). Imaging modalities used to distinguish between these entities include CT-PET, MR spectroscopy, MR diffusion, and MR perfusion. However, none of these techniques are yet definitive and clinical judgement and close imaging surveillance are indicated [91]. Radiation necrosis may occur in up to 50% of brain metastases treated with SRS [92–95], the risk increasing with larger target volume and fraction dose [92, 96]. Changes may become evident on imaging 3 months to 3 years following treatment, with a peak around 11 months. Pathological features include thrombosis and haemorrhage, fibrinous exudates and vascular fibrosis/hyalinization with luminal stenosis and occlusion. Congealed, fibrin-rich areas of gliosis contain dystrophic calcifications and macrophage infiltration. Excess extracellular proteolysis promotes cytokine activation and cytotoxic oedema, and other immune-mediated mechanisms may contribute to radiation-induced neurotoxicity [97].

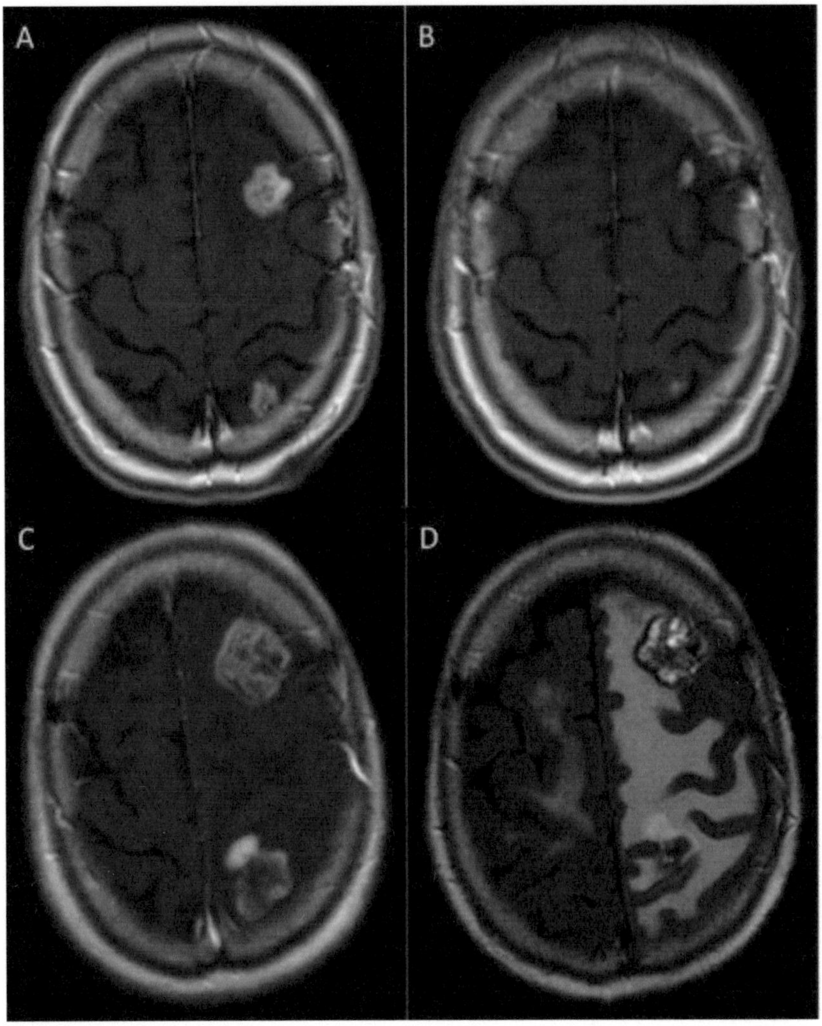

Figure 4. (A) Pre-treatment gadolinium contrast-enhanced T1 MRI showing two left-sided metastases. (B) Gadolinium contrast-enhanced T1 MRI showing decrease in lesion size after treatment. (C) T1 gadolinium contrast-enhanced and (D) T2 MRI 10 months after treatment, showing increase in enhancing lesion size and peri-lesional oedema.

The mainstay of treatment for symptomatic radiation necrosis is corticosteroids continued at the lowest effective dose until symptoms resolve [98]. In patients who develop adverse effects or are unable to tolerate corticosteroids, a small randomised placebo-controlled trial and some retrospective studies have shown that bevacizumab can be effective in reducing cerebral oedema and neurologic symptoms associated with radiation necrosis, as well as FLAIR and enhancement changes seen on MRI [99, 100]. While bevacizumab can markedly improve symptoms and imaging, adverse effects may include intracranial haemorrhage and wound healing complications should surgery become necessary, and careful patient selection is necessary [101]. In addition, several case reports and small series have suggested that hyperbaric oxygen (HBO) can also have a role in treatment of intracerebral radiation necrosis, with improvement in neurologic symptoms, decreased steroid requirement and reduced lesion size on imaging [102, 103].

Surgical resection should be considered in patients refractory or intolerant to corticosteroids, if the radiation necrosis has significant mass effect, or if imaging is equivocal and tumour progression remains a concern. If a lesion is not safely accessible, a biopsy may be considered to rule out active disease.

In this case, oedema causing mass effect and headaches can be treated with corticosteroids. As the diagnosis is uncertain, repeat imaging and clinical follow-up should be carried out in a short interval.

Case 5: Molecular profiling and targeted therapy

A 63-year-old man presents to the emergency department for evaluation following a motor vehicle collision. A single 6-mm lesion is identified in the right posterior midbrain, which demonstrates ring-enhancement on MRI (Figure 5). The patient's past medical history is significant for melanoma treated with surgical excision 15 years prior.

In a patient who has undergone treatment for a cancer with a propensity for intracranial dissemination, a new brain lesion may be a metastatic deposit. However, in patients with a known primary malignancy, 11% may have a solitary brain lesion that is not metastatic [33]. Current imaging modalities have greatly improved the specificity of distinguishing brain metastases from primary tumours and other pathologies [104–106], but diagnostic certainty is essential to appropriate treatment planning and prognostication. In addition, some primary histologies include molecular subtypes that can benefit from targeted therapy, and patients who underwent diagnosis and treatment prior to the routine molecular profiling of such tumours may yet benefit from updated pathological analysis.

In melanoma containing the *BRAF* V600E mutation, the BRAF inhibitors dabrafenib [89] and vemurafenib [107] have demonstrated effect against brain metastases. The receptor tyrosine kinase inhibitors erlotinib and gefitinib show effect in NSCLC with an EGFR mutation [76], and crizotinib has shown some activity against NSCLC containing *ALK* rearrangement [79]. Furthermore, an alteration in oestrogen receptor (ER), progesterone receptor (PR) and HER2 expression between primary and metastatic deposits is observed in >10% of breast cancers, requiring an alteration in management [108]. In patients who have HER2-postive tumours, a phase II trial demonstrated a 66% rate of objective CNS response for the combination of lapatinib and capecitabine [86].

In this case, the long latency period since the patient's initial cancer presentation warrants histologic diagnosis of the cerebral lesion. In a deep location, needle biopsy would allow for safe extraction of diagnostic tissue.

Case 6: Prognostic considerations

A 78-year-old man who resides in a nursing home due to memory impairment undergoes evaluation for recurrent falls. MRI of the brain demonstrates atrophy and white matter

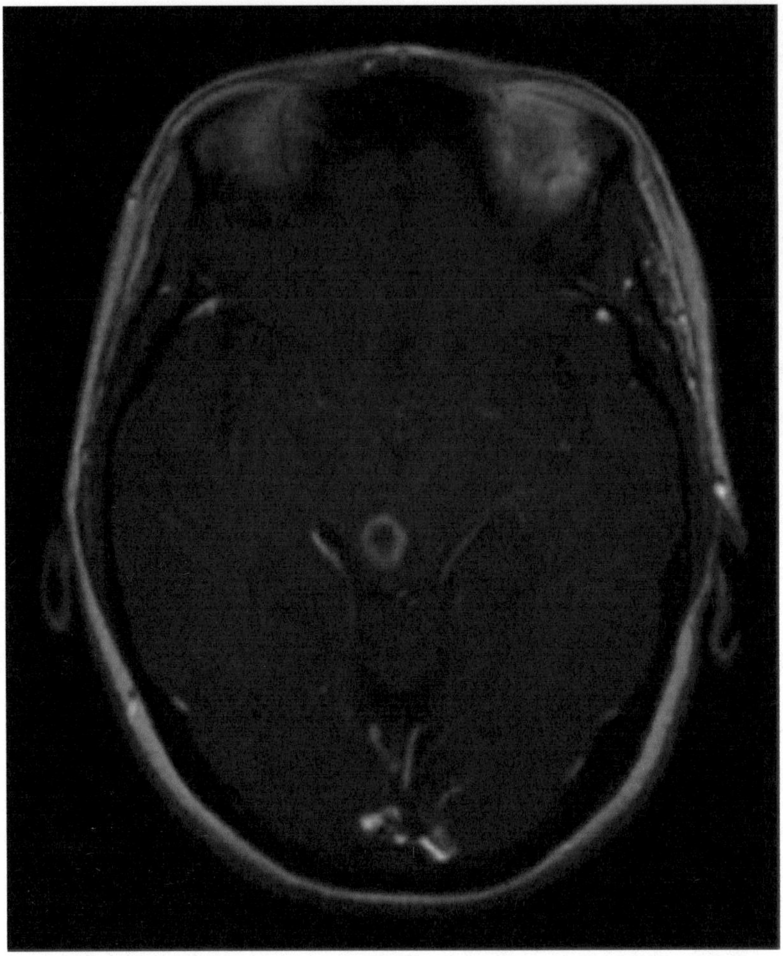

Figure 5. Gadolinium contrast-enhanced T1 MRI of incidentally found midbrain lesion.

changes as well as numerous enhancing lesions suggestive of metastatic deposits (Figure 6). Systemic work-up reveals a rectal mass, as well as extensive retroperitoneal lymphadenopathy and a hepatic lesion, consistent with metastatic colorectal carcinoma.

The RTOG recursive partitioning analysis (RPA) identified Karnofsky performance status (KPS) as a key prognostic factor in patients with brain metastases [18]. The diagnosis-specific graded prognostic assessment found that certain RPA factors were not significant for some primary histologies, but KPS retained significance in all diagnoses [109]. In a patient with poor functional status, aggressive treatment of brain metastases is not indicated due to a short expected survival. WBRT may be offered to palliate neurological symptoms caused by intracerebral lesions and associated oedema. A radiographic response is seen in 40–60% of patients, with neurologic improvement in 25–40% [25, 52]. Observational studies suggest

http://dx.doi.org/10.5772/66310

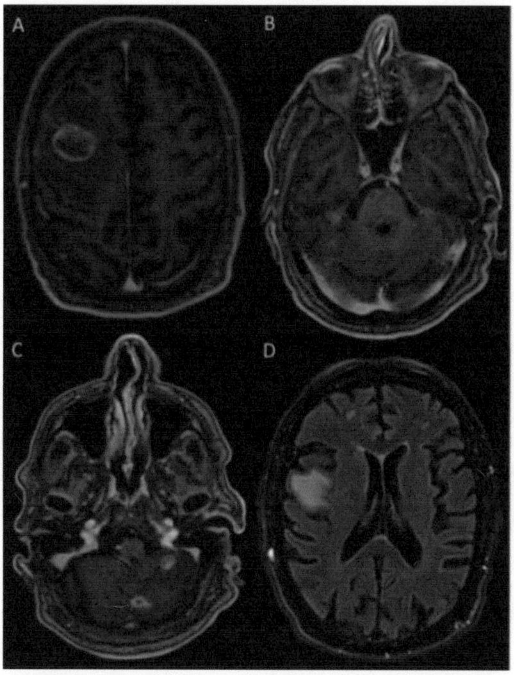

Figure 6. (A)–(C) T1 gadolinium contrast-enhanced MRI demonstrating cerebral atrophy and multiple metastases. (D) FLAIR sequence showing white-matter changes distinct from enhancing lesions.

an improvement in survival compared to corticosteroids/supportive therapy [110, 111]. However, radiotherapy requires daily treatment sessions for 10–15 days, and acute radiation toxicity may cause fatigue, nausea, vomiting, anorexia, alopecia, and radiation dermatitis [112]. Where numerous repeat treatments are not feasible, a single fraction of 6–8 Gy may be considered, accepting a lower rate of tumour control and possibly greater acute toxicity. Alternatively, in patients with poor medical and/or functional status, supportive care alone may be the most appropriate management.

In this case, without focal neurologic deficits, limited intervention with a focus on patient comfort is a reasonable approach.

5. Conclusion

The brain is a common site of progression for patients with cancer, and brain metastases are associated with significant morbidity and mortality. Many modalities of treatment are available aimed at controlling neurologic progression and overall survival, as well as palliating symptoms. A thoroughly multidisciplinary approach is therefore required for comprehensive and effective management of brain metastases.

Author details

Karolyn Au[1,*], Ying Meng[1], Suganth Suppiah[1], Anick Nater[1], Rakesh Jalali[2] and Gelareh Zadeh[1]

*Address all correspondence to: karolyn@ualberta.ca

1 Toronto Western Hospital, University of Toronto, Toronto, Canada

2 Tata Memorial Centre, Mumbai, India

References

[1] Tabouret E, Chinot O, Metellus P, Tallet A, Viens P, Goncalves A. Recent trends in epidemiology of brain metastases: an overview. Anticancer Res. 2012;32(11):4655–62.

[2] Nayak L, Lee EQ, Wen PY. Epidemiology of brain metastases. Curr Oncol Rep. 2012; 14(1):48–54.

[3] Taillibert S, Le Rhun E. [Epidemiology of brain metastases]. Cancer Radiother. 2015; 19(1):3–9.

[4] Langer CJ, Mehta MP. Current management of brain metastases, with a focus on systemic options. J Clin Oncol. 2005;23(25):6207–19.

[5] Fox BD, Cheung VJ, Patel AJ, Suki D, Rao G. Epidemiology of metastatic brain tumors. Neurosurg Clin N Am. 2011;22(1):1–6.

[6] Barnholtz-Sloan JS, Sloan AE, Davis FG, Vigneau FD, Lai P, Sawaya RE. Incidence proportions of brain metastases in patients diagnosed (1973 to 2001) in the Metropolitan Detroit Cancer Surveillance System. J Clin Oncol. 2004;22(14):2865–72.

[7] Schouten LJ, Rutten J, Huveneers HA, Twijnstra A. Incidence of brain metastases in a cohort of patients with carcinoma of the breast, colon, kidney, and lung and melanoma. Cancer. 2002;94(10):2698–705.

[8] Chason JL, Walker FB, Landers JW. Metastatic carcinoma in the central nervous system and dorsal root ganglia. A prospective autopsy study. Cancer. 1963;16:781–7.

[9] Posner JB, Chernik NL. Intracranial metastases from systemic cancer. Adv Neurol. 1978;19:579–92.

[10] Smedby KE, Brandt L, Backlund ML, Blomqvist P. Brain metastases admissions in Sweden between 1987 and 2006. Br J Cancer. 2009;101(11):1919–24.

[11] Siegel R, Ma J, Zou Z, Jemal A. Cancer statistics, 2014. CA Cancer J Clin. 2014;64(1):9–29.

[12] Schootman M, Jeffe DB, Gillanders WE, Aft R. Racial disparities in the development of breast cancer metastases among older women: a multilevel study. Cancer. 2009;115(4):731–40.

[13] Lagerwaard FJ, Levendag PC, Nowak PJ, Eijkenboom WM, Hanssens PE, Schmitz PI. Identification of prognostic factors in patients with brain metastases: a review of 1292 patients. Int J Radiat Oncol Biol Phys. 1999;43(4):795–803.

[14] Nussbaum ES, Djalilian HR, Cho KH, Hall WA. Brain metastases. Histology, multiplicity, surgery, and survival. Cancer. 1996;78(8):1781–8.

[15] Stark AM, Stohring C, Hedderich J, Held-Feindt J, Mehdorn HM. Surgical treatment for brain metastases: Prognostic factors and survival in 309 patients with regard to patient age. J Clin Neurosci. 2011;18(1):34–8.

[16] Yawn BP, Wollan PC, Schroeder C, Gazzuola L, Mehta M. Temporal and gender-related trends in brain metastases from lung and breast cancer. Minn Med. 2003;86(12):32–7.

[17] Nieder C, Spanne O, Mehta MP, Grosu AL, Geinitz H. Presentation, patterns of care, and survival in patients with brain metastases: what has changed in the last 20 years? Cancer. 2011;117(11):2505–12.

[18] Gaspar L, Scott C, Rotman M, Asbell S, Phillips T, Wasserman T, et al. Recursive partitioning analysis (RPA) of prognostic factors in three Radiation Therapy Oncology Group (RTOG) brain metastases trials. Int J Radiat Oncol Biol Phys. 1997;37(4):745–51.

[19] Fabi A, Felici A, Metro G, Mirri A, Bria E, Telera S, et al. Brain metastases from solid tumors: disease outcome according to type of treatment and therapeutic resources of the treating center. J Exp Clin Cancer Res. 2011;30:10.

[20] Sperduto PW, Kased N, Roberge D, Xu Z, Shanley R, Luo X, et al. Summary report on the graded prognostic assessment: an accurate and facile diagnosis-specific tool to estimate survival for patients with brain metastases. J Clin Oncol. 2012;30(4):419–25.

[21] Zhang X, Zhang W, Cao WD, Cheng G, Liu B, Cheng J. A review of current management of brain metastases. Ann Surg Oncol. 2012;19(3):1043–50.

[22] Gaspar LE, Mehta MP, Patchell RA, Burri SH, Robinson PD, Morris RE, et al. The role of whole brain radiation therapy in the management of newly diagnosed brain metastases: a systematic review and evidence-based clinical practice guideline. J Neurooncol. 2010;96(1):17–32.

[23] Soffietti R, Ruda R, Mutani R. Management of brain metastases. J Neurol. 2002;249 (10):1357–69.

[24] DeAngelis LM. Management of brain metastases. Cancer Invest. 1994;12(2):156–65.

[25] Borgelt B, Gelber R, Kramer S, Brady LW, Chang CH, Davis LW, et al. The palliation of brain metastases: final results of the first two studies by the Radiation Therapy Oncology Group. Int J Radiat Oncol Biol Phys. 1980;6(1):1–9.

[26] Kurtz JM, Gelber R, Brady LW, Carella RJ, Cooper JS. The palliation of brain metastases in a favorable patient population: a randomized clinical trial by the Radiation Therapy Oncology Group. Int J Radiat Oncol Biol Phys. 1981;7(7):891–5.

[27] DeAngelis LM, Delattre JY, Posner JB. Radiation-induced dementia in patients cured of brain metastases. Neurology. 1989;39(6):789–96.

[28] Sun A, Bae K, Gore EM, Movsas B, Wong SJ, Meyers CA, et al. Phase III trial of prophylactic cranial irradiation compared with observation in patients with locally advanced non-small-cell lung cancer: neurocognitive and quality-of-life analysis. J Clin Oncol. 2011;29(3):279–86.

[29] Komaki R, Meyers CA, Shin DM, Garden AS, Byrne K, Nickens JA, et al. Evaluation of cognitive function in patients with limited small cell lung cancer prior to and shortly following prophylactic cranial irradiation. Int J Radiat Oncol Biol Phys. 1995;33(1):179–82.

[30] Regine WF, Scott C, Murray K, Curran W. Neurocognitive outcome in brain metastases patients treated with accelerated-fractionation vs. accelerated-hyperfractionated radiotherapy: an analysis from Radiation Therapy Oncology Group Study 91–04. Int J Radiat Oncol Biol Phys. 2001;51(3):711–7.

[31] Gondi V, Pugh SL, Tome WA, Caine C, Corn B, Kanner A, et al. Preservation of memory with conformal avoidance of the hippocampal neural stem-cell compartment during whole-brain radiotherapy for brain metastases (RTOG 0933): a phase II multi-institutional trial. J Clin Oncol. 2014;32(34):3810–6.

[32] Brown PD, Pugh S, Laack NN, Wefel JS, Khuntia D, Meyers C, et al. Memantine for the prevention of cognitive dysfunction in patients receiving whole-brain radiotherapy: a randomized, double-blind, placebo-controlled trial. Neuro Oncol. 2013;15(10):1429–37.

[33] Patchell RA, Tibbs PA, Walsh JW, Dempsey RJ, Maruyama Y, Kryscio RJ, et al. A randomized trial of surgery in the treatment of single metastases to the brain. N Engl J Med. 1990;322(8):494–500.

[34] Vecht CJ, Haaxma-Reiche H, Noordijk EM, Padberg GW, Voormolen JH, Hoekstra FH, et al. Treatment of single brain metastasis: radiotherapy alone or combined with neurosurgery? Ann Neurol. 1993;33(6):583–90.

[35] Mintz AH, Kestle J, Rathbone MP, Gaspar L, Hugenholtz H, Fisher B, et al. A randomized trial to assess the efficacy of surgery in addition to radiotherapy in patients with a single cerebral metastasis. Cancer. 1996;78(7):1470–6.

[36] Bindal RK, Sawaya R, Leavens ME, Lee JJ. Surgical treatment of multiple brain metastases. J Neurosurg. 1993;79(2):210–6.

[37] Paek SH, Audu PB, Sperling MR, Cho J, Andrews DW. Reevaluation of surgery for the treatment of brain metastases: review of 208 patients with single or multiple brain metastases treated at one institution with modern neurosurgical techniques. Neurosurgery. 2005;56(5):1021–34; discussion 1021–34.

[38] Iwadate Y, Namba H, Yamaura A. Significance of surgical resection for the treatment of multiple brain metastases. Anticancer Res. 2000;20(1B):573–7.

[39] Armstrong JG, Wronski M, Galicich J, Arbit E, Leibel SA, Burt M. Postoperative radiation for lung cancer metastatic to the brain. J Clin Oncol. 1994;12(11):2340–4.

[40] Hagen NA, Cirrincione C, Thaler HT, DeAngelis LM. The role of radiation therapy following resection of single brain metastasis from melanoma. Neurology. 1990;40(1):158–60.

[41] DeAngelis LM, Mandell LR, Thaler HT, Kimmel DW, Galicich JH, Fuks Z, et al. The role of postoperative radiotherapy after resection of single brain metastases. Neurosurgery. 1989;24(6):798–805.

[42] Patchell RA, Tibbs PA, Regine WF, Dempsey RJ, Mohiuddin M, Kryscio RJ, et al. Postoperative radiotherapy in the treatment of single metastases to the brain: a randomized trial. JAMA. 1998;280(17):1485–9.

[43] Kocher M, Soffietti R, Abacioglu U, Villa S, Fauchon F, Baumert BG, et al. Adjuvant whole-brain radiotherapy versus observation after radiosurgery or surgical resection of one to three cerebral metastases: results of the EORTC 22952–26001 study. J Clin Oncol. 2011;29(2):134–41.

[44] Mathieu D, Kondziolka D, Flickinger JC, Fortin D, Kenny B, Michaud K, et al. Tumor bed radiosurgery after resection of cerebral metastases. Neurosurgery. 2008;62(4):817–23; discussion 23–4.

[45] Soltys SG, Adler JR, Lipani JD, Jackson PS, Choi CY, Puataweepong P, et al. Stereotactic radiosurgery of the postoperative resection cavity for brain metastases. Int J Radiat Oncol Biol Phys. 2008;70(1):187–93.

[46] Hwang SW, Abozed MM, Hale A, Eisenberg RL, Dvorak T, Yao K, et al. Adjuvant Gamma Knife radiosurgery following surgical resection of brain metastases: a 9-year retrospective cohort study. J Neurooncol. 2010;98(1):77–82.

[47] Brennan C, Yang TJ, Hilden P, Zhang Z, Chan K, Yamada Y, et al. A phase 2 trial of stereotactic radiosurgery boost after surgical resection for brain metastases. Int J Radiat Oncol Biol Phys. 2014;88(1):130–6.

[48] Shiau CY, Sneed PK, Shu HK, Lamborn KR, McDermott MW, Chang S, et al. Radiosurgery for brain metastases: relationship of dose and pattern of enhancement to local control. Int J Radiat Oncol Biol Phys. 1997;37(2):375–83.

[49] Sneed PK, Mendez J, Vemer-van den Hoek JG, Seymour ZA, Ma L, Molinaro AM, et al. Adverse radiation effect after stereotactic radiosurgery for brain metastases: incidence, time course, and risk factors. J Neurosurg. 2015;123(2):373–86.

[50] Parvez K, Parvez A, Zadeh G. The diagnosis and treatment of pseudoprogression, radiation necrosis and brain tumor recurrence. Int J Mol Sci. 2014;15(7):11832–46.

[51] Kondziolka D, Patel A, Lunsford LD, Kassam A, Flickinger JC. Stereotactic radiosurgery plus whole brain radiotherapy versus radiotherapy alone for patients with multiple brain metastases. Int J Radiat Oncol Biol Phys. 1999;45(2):427–34.

[52] Andrews DW, Scott CB, Sperduto PW, Flanders AE, Gaspar LE, Schell MC, et al. Whole brain radiation therapy with or without stereotactic radiosurgery boost for patients with one to three brain metastases: phase III results of the RTOG 9508 randomised trial. Lancet. 2004;363(9422):1665–72.

[53] Sperduto PW, Shanley R, Luo X, Andrews D, Werner-Wasik M, Valicenti R, et al. Secondary analysis of RTOG 9508, a phase 3 randomized trial of whole-brain radiation therapy versus WBRT plus stereotactic radiosurgery in patients with 1–3 brain metastases; poststratified by the graded prognostic assessment (GPA). Int J Radiat Oncol Biol Phys. 2014;90(3):526–31.

[54] O'Neill BP, Iturria NJ, Link MJ, Pollock BE, Ballman KV, O'Fallon JR. A comparison of surgical resection and stereotactic radiosurgery in the treatment of solitary brain metastases. Int J Radiat Oncol Biol Phys. 2003;55(5):1169–76.

[55] Schoggl A, Kitz K, Reddy M, Wolfsberger S, Schneider B, Dieckmann K, et al. Defining the role of stereotactic radiosurgery versus microsurgery in the treatment of single brain metastases. Acta Neurochir (Wien). 2000;142(6):621–6.

[56] Bindal AK, Bindal RK, Hess KR, Shiu A, Hassenbusch SJ, Shi WM, et al. Surgery versus radiosurgery in the treatment of brain metastasis. J Neurosurg. 1996;84(5):748–54.

[57] Auchter RM, Lamond JP, Alexander E, Buatti JM, Chappell R, Friedman WA, et al. A multiinstitutional outcome and prognostic factor analysis of radiosurgery for resectable single brain metastasis. Int J Radiat Oncol Biol Phys. 1996;35(1):27–35.

[58] Muacevic A, Wowra B, Siefert A, Tonn JC, Steiger HJ, Kreth FW. Microsurgery plus whole brain irradiation versus Gamma Knife surgery alone for treatment of single metastases to the brain: a randomized controlled multicentre phase III trial. J Neurooncol. 2008;87(3):299–307.

[59] Aoyama H, Shirato H, Tago M, Nakagawa K, Toyoda T, Hatano K, et al. Stereotactic radiosurgery plus whole-brain radiation therapy vs stereotactic radiosurgery alone for treatment of brain metastases: a randomized controlled trial. JAMA. 2006;295(21):2483–91.

[60] Chang EL, Wefel JS, Hess KR, Allen PK, Lang FF, Kornguth DG, et al. Neurocognition in patients with brain metastases treated with radiosurgery or radiosurgery plus whole-brain irradiation: a randomised controlled trial. Lancet Oncol. 2009;10(11):1037–44.

[61] Brown PD, Jaeckle K, Ballman KV, Farace E, Cerhan JH, Anderson SK, et al. Effect of radiosurgery alone vs radiosurgery with whole brain radiation therapy on cognitive function in patients with 1 to 3 brain metastases: A randomized clinical Trial. JAMA. 2016;316(4):401–9.

[62] Yamamoto M, Serizawa T, Shuto T, Akabane A, Higuchi Y, Kawagishi J, et al. Stereotactic radiosurgery for patients with multiple brain metastases (JLGK0901): a multi-institutional prospective observational study. Lancet Oncol. 2014;15(4):387–95.

[63] Chao ST, Barnett GH, Vogelbaum MA, Angelov L, Weil RJ, Neyman G, et al. Salvage stereotactic radiosurgery effectively treats recurrences from whole-brain radiation therapy. Cancer. 2008;113(8):2198–204.

[64] Kurtz G, Zadeh G, Gingras-Hill G, Millar BA, Laperriere NJ, Bernstein M, et al. Salvage radiosurgery for brain metastases: prognostic factors to consider in patient selection. Int J Radiat Oncol Biol Phys. 2014;88(1):137–42.

[65] Minniti G, Scaringi C, Paolini S, Clarke E, Cicone F, Esposito V, et al. Repeated stereotactic radiosurgery for patients with progressive brain metastases. J Neurooncol. 2016;126(1):91–7.

[66] Lalondrelle S, Khoo V. Brain metastases. BMJ Clin Evid. 2009;2009:1018.

[67] Christodoulou C, Bafaloukos D, Kosmidis P, Samantas E, Bamias A, Papakostas P, et al. Phase II study of temozolomide in heavily pretreated cancer patients with brain metastases. Ann Oncol. 2001;12(2):249–54.

[68] Abrey LE, Olson JD, Raizer JJ, Mack M, Rodavitch A, Boutros DY, et al. A phase II trial of temozolomide for patients with recurrent or progressive brain metastases. J Neurooncol. 2001;53(3):259–65.

[69] Zhu W, Zhou L, Qian JQ, Qiu TZ, Shu YQ, Liu P. Temozolomide for treatment of brain metastases: A review of 21 clinical trials. World J Clin Oncol. 2014;5(1):19–27.

[70] Grossi F, Scolaro T, Tixi L, Loprevite M, Ardizzoni A. The role of systemic chemotherapy in the treatment of brain metastases from small-cell lung cancer. Crit Rev Oncol Hematol. 2001;37(1):61–7.

[71] Kaal EC, Niel CG, Vecht CJ. Therapeutic management of brain metastasis. Lancet Neurol. 2005;4(5):289–98.

[72] Eichler AF, Loeffler JS. Multidisciplinary management of brain metastases. Oncologist. 2007;12(7):884–98.

[73] Chiu CH, Tsai CM, Chen YM, Chiang SC, Liou JL, Perng RP. Gefitinib is active in patients with brain metastases from non-small cell lung cancer and response is related to skin toxicity. Lung Cancer. 2005;47(1):129–38.

[74] Kim JE, Lee DH, Choi Y, Yoon DH, Kim SW, Suh C, et al. Epidermal growth factor receptor tyrosine kinase inhibitors as a first-line therapy for never-smokers with adenocarcinoma of the lung having asymptomatic synchronous brain metastasis. Lung Cancer. 2009;65(3):351–4.

[75] Porta R, Sanchez-Torres JM, Paz-Ares L, Massuti B, Reguart N, Mayo C, et al. Brain metastases from lung cancer responding to erlotinib: the importance of EGFR mutation. Eur Respir J. 2011;37(3):624–31.

[76] Jamal-Hanjani M, Spicer J. Epidermal growth factor receptor tyrosine kinase inhibitors in the treatment of epidermal growth factor receptor-mutant non-small cell lung cancer metastatic to the brain. Clin Cancer Res. 2012;18(4):938–44.

[77] Wu YL, Zhou C, Cheng Y, Lu S, Chen GY, Huang C, et al. Erlotinib as second-line treatment in patients with advanced non-small-cell lung cancer and asymptomatic brain metastases: a phase II study (CTONG-0803). Ann Oncol. 2013;24(4):993–9.

[78] Doebele RC, Lu X, Sumey C, Maxson DA, Weickhardt AJ, Oton AB, et al. Oncogene status predicts patterns of metastatic spread in treatment-naive nonsmall cell lung cancer. Cancer. 2012;118(18):4502–11.

[79] Costa DB, Shaw AT, Ou SH, Solomon BJ, Riely GJ, Ahn MJ, et al. Clinical experience with crizotinib in patients with advanced ALK-rearranged non-small-cell lung cancer and brain metastases. J Clin Oncol. 2015;33(17):1881–8.

[80] Rusthoven CG, Doebele RC. Management of brain metastases in ALK-positive non-small-cell lung cancer. J Clin Oncol. 2016;34(24):2814–9.

[81] Jiang T, Min W, Li Y, Yue Z, Wu C, Zhou C. Radiotherapy plus EGFR TKIs in non-small cell lung cancer patients with brain metastases: an update meta-analysis. Cancer Med. 2016;5(6):1055–65.

[82] Lim E, Lin NU. Updates on the management of breast cancer brain metastases. Oncology (Williston Park). 2014;28(7):572–8.

[83] Yin W, Jiang Y, Shen Z, Shao Z, Lu J. Trastuzumab in the adjuvant treatment of HER2-positive early breast cancer patients: a meta-analysis of published randomized controlled trials. PLoS One. 2011;6(6):e21030.

[84] Lin NU, Dieras V, Paul D, Lossignol D, Christodoulou C, Stemmler HJ, et al. Multicenter phase II study of lapatinib in patients with brain metastases from HER2-positive breast cancer. Clin Cancer Res. 2009;15(4):1452–9.

[85] Lin NU, Carey LA, Liu MC, Younger J, Come SE, Ewend M, et al. Phase II trial of lapatinib for brain metastases in patients with human epidermal growth factor receptor 2-positive breast cancer. J Clin Oncol. 2008;26(12):1993–9.

[86] Bachelot T, Romieu G, Campone M, Dieras V, Cropet C, Dalenc F, et al. Lapatinib plus capecitabine in patients with previously untreated brain metastases from HER2-positive metastatic breast cancer (LANDSCAPE): a single-group phase 2 study. Lancet Oncol. 2013;14(1):64–71.

[87] Margolin K, Ernstoff MS, Hamid O, Lawrence D, McDermott D, Puzanov I, et al. Ipilimumab in patients with melanoma and brain metastases: an open-label, phase 2 trial. Lancet Oncol. 2012;13(5):459–65.

[88] Tazi K, Hathaway A, Chiuzan C, Shirai K. Survival of melanoma patients with brain metastases treated with ipilimumab and stereotactic radiosurgery. Cancer Med. 2015;4(1):1–6.

[89] Long GV, Trefzer U, Davies MA, Kefford RF, Ascierto PA, Chapman PB, et al. Dabrafenib in patients with Val600Glu or Val600Lys BRAF-mutant melanoma metastatic to the brain (BREAK-MB): a multicentre, open-label, phase 2 trial. Lancet Oncol. 2012;13(11):1087–95.

[90] Soon YY, Tham IW, Lim KH, Koh WY, Lu JJ. Surgery or radiosurgery plus whole brain radiotherapy versus surgery or radiosurgery alone for brain metastases. Cochrane Database Syst Rev. 2014;3:CD009454.

[91] Lin NU, Lee EQ, Aoyama H, Barani IJ, Barboriak DP, Baumert BG, et al. Response assessment criteria for brain metastases: proposal from the RANO group. Lancet Oncol. 2015;16(6):e270–8.

[92] Blonigen BJ, Steinmetz RD, Levin L, Lamba MA, Warnick RE, Breneman JC. Irradiated volume as a predictor of brain radionecrosis after linear accelerator stereotactic radiosurgery. Int J Radiat Oncol Biol Phys. 2010;77(4):996–1001.

[93] Shaw E, Scott C, Souhami L, Dinapoli R, Kline R, Loeffler J, et al. Single dose radiosurgical treatment of recurrent previously irradiated primary brain tumors and brain metastases: final report of RTOG protocol 90–05. Int J Radiat Oncol Biol Phys. 2000;47(2):291–8.

[94] Voges J, Treuer H, Sturm V, Buchner C, Lehrke R, Kocher M, et al. Risk analysis of linear accelerator radiosurgery. Int J Radiat Oncol Biol Phys. 1996;36(5):1055–63.

[95] Petrovich Z, Yu C, Giannotta SL, O'Day S, Apuzzo ML. Survival and pattern of failure in brain metastasis treated with stereotactic gamma knife radiosurgery. J Neurosurg. 2002;97(Suppl 5):499–506.

[96] Minniti G, Clarke E, Lanzetta G, Osti MF, Trasimeni G, Bozzao A, et al. Stereotactic radiosurgery for brain metastases: analysis of outcome and risk of brain radionecrosis. Radiat Oncol. 2011;6:48.

[97] Perry A, Schmidt RE. Cancer therapy-associated CNS neuropathology: an update and review of the literature. Acta Neuropathol. 2006;111(3):197–212.

[98] Shaw PJ, Bates D. Conservative treatment of delayed cerebral radiation necrosis. J Neurol Neurosurg Psychiatry. 1984;47(12):1338–41.

[99] Levin VA, Bidaut L, Hou P, Kumar AJ, Wefel JS, Bekele BN, et al. Randomized double-blind placebo-controlled trial of bevacizumab therapy for radiation necrosis of the central nervous system. Int J Radiat Oncol Biol Phys. 2011;79(5):1487–95.

[100] Sadraei NH, Dahiya S, Chao ST, Murphy ES, Osei-Boateng K, Xie H, et al. Treatment of cerebral radiation necrosis with bevacizumab: the Cleveland clinic experience. Am J Clin Oncol. 2015;38(3):304–10.

[101] Narita Y. Drug review: Safety and efficacy of bevacizumab for glioblastoma and other brain tumors. Jpn J Clin Oncol. 2013;43(6):587–95.

[102] Kohshi K, Imada H, Nomoto S, Yamaguchi R, Abe H, Yamamoto H. Successful treatment of radiation-induced brain necrosis by hyperbaric oxygen therapy. J Neurol Sci. 2003;209(1–2):115–7.

[103] Leber KA, Eder HG, Kovac H, Anegg U, Pendl G. Treatment of cerebral radionecrosis by hyperbaric oxygen therapy. Stereotact Funct Neurosurg. 1998;70(Suppl 1):229–36.

[104] Fink KR, Fink JR. Imaging of brain metastases. Surg Neurol Int. 2013;4(Suppl 4):S209–19.

[105] Ding Y, Xing Z, Liu B, Lin X, Cao D. Differentiation of primary central nervous system lymphoma from high-grade glioma and brain metastases using susceptibility-weighted imaging. Brain Behav. 2014;4(6):841–9.

[106] Wang S, Kim S, Chawla S, Wolf RL, Knipp DE, Vossough A, et al. Differentiation between glioblastomas, solitary brain metastases, and primary cerebral lymphomas using diffusion tensor and dynamic susceptibility contrast-enhanced MR imaging. AJNR Am J Neuroradiol. 2011;32(3):507–14.

[107] Harding JJ, Catalanotti F, Munhoz RR, Cheng DT, Yaqubie A, Kelly N, et al. A retrospective evaluation of vemurafenib as treatment for BRAF-mutant melanoma brain metastases. Oncologist. 2015;20(7):789–97.

[108] Amir E, Miller N, Geddie W, Freedman O, Kassam F, Simmons C, et al. Prospective study evaluating the impact of tissue confirmation of metastatic disease in patients with breast cancer. J Clin Oncol. 2012;30(6):587–92.

[109] Sperduto PW, Chao ST, Sneed PK, Luo X, Suh J, Roberge D, et al. Diagnosis-specific prognostic factors, indexes, and treatment outcomes for patients with newly diagnosed brain metastases: a multi-institutional analysis of 4,259 patients. Int J Radiat Oncol Biol Phys. 2010;77(3):655–61.

[110] Zimm S, Wampler GL, Stablein D, Hazra T, Young HF. Intracerebral metastases in solid-tumor patients: natural history and results of treatment. Cancer. 1981;48(2):384–94.

[111] Sneed PK, Larson DA, Wara WM. Radiotherapy for cerebral metastases. Neurosurg Clin N Am. 1996;7(3):505–15.

[112] Cross NE, Glantz MJ. Neurologic complications of radiation therapy. Neurol Clin. 2003;21(1):249–77.

Chapter 7

Advances in the Treatment of Primary Brain Tumors: The Realm of Immunotherapy

Michael J. Strong and Marcus L. Ware

Additional information is available at the end of the chapter

http://dx.doi.org/10.5772/64611

Abstract

Central nervous system (CNS) tumors, although rare, represent a group of neoplasms that have a disproportionate morbidity and mortality. Despite advances in our understanding of tumor pathogenesis coupled with improvements in therapeutic options, overall survival for primary brain tumors remains dismal. Although challenging, newer approaches such as brachytherapy, immunotherapy, and electric field generators are currently being evaluated in the clinical setting with promising results. The field of immunotherapy in neurooncology is still in its infancy, but several advances have already been made, including the development of tumor vaccines, utilization of immune checkpoint inhibitors, and activation of tumor dendritic cells to stimulate the host's immune system. Recent advances in noninvasive electric fields have been applied to the treatment of glioblastoma multiforme (GBM) with encouraging clinical outcome. In this chapter, we will review the latest advances in the treatment of glioblastoma multiforme with a focus on immunotherapy.

Keywords: glioblastomas, immunotherapy, tumor vaccines, immune checkpoint inhibitors, tumor treating fields

1. Introduction

Central nervous system (CNS) tumors comprise a relatively small portion of cancers, but they are among the most aggressive tumors and result in significant morbidity and mortality. It is estimated that approximately 77,670 cases of primary CNS tumors are expected to be diagnosed in the United States in 2016 [1]. Of these, roughly 40% will be malignant with the majority being glioblastoma multiforme (GBM). The median survival of newly diagnosed subjects with GBM is approximately 12–15 months [2]. Despite intense efforts into understanding disease mechanisms and advances in technology, overall survival has only improved by

3–6 months, and the 5-year survival rate ranks sixth lowest among all cancers after pancreatic, liver, intrahepatic bile duct, lung, stomach, and esophageal [3, 4].

Traditional treatment approaches for brain tumors have relied upon a combination of surgical resection, radiation, and chemotherapy. Newer approaches such as brachytherapy, immunotherapy, and electric field generators are currently being evaluated in the clinical setting. In this chapter, we review the latest advances in the treatment of GBM.

2. Gliomas

Gliomas are the most common primary malignant brain tumor, comprising more than 80% of all malignant brain neoplasms [5]. Gliomas can be further divided into astrocytomas, oligodendrogliomas, ependymomas, and mixed gliomas (i.e., oligoastrocytomas). These tumors can be further characterized based on grading. Astrocytomas are graded from I through IV and are represented as follows: grade I—pilocytic, grade II—diffuse, grade III—anaplastic, and grade IV—glioblastoma multiforme (GBM). Although we historically call all grade IV astrocytomas GBM and subsequently treat these tumors with the same treatment protocols, growing evidence suggests that even within GBM, there may be distinct disease processes that require a more specific targeting approach. Recently, GBM was re-classified into four subtypes based on unique molecular profiles and includes: classical, mesenchymal, proneural, and neural [6]. Further analysis of these subtypes identified subjects with classical GBMs lived the longest compared to those subjects with other GBM subtypes [6]. This observation may partly explain some subjects with GBM having lengthened overall survival compared to other GBM subjects.

Subjects with CNS tumors may present with any generalized or focal symptoms including a headache, seizure, or a specific neurological deficit. However, one of the most common complaints for CNS tumor subjects is a headache with roughly 77% of subjects reporting a dull tension-like headache [7]. Seizures are also very common in CNS tumor subjects with roughly 15–95% of subjects experiencing at least one seizure during the course of their disease process [8]. Interestingly, seizures are more common in subjects aged 30–50 years and are frequently associated with tumors involving the frontal, temporal, frontotemporal, and frontoparietal lobes [9].

Due to the relatively rapid natural progression of GBM, identification of prognostic factors is valuable in determining the most appropriate therapeutic approach for subjects. Traditional indicators used include subject's age, their Karnofsky performance score, tumor size and location, and finally grade of tumor. In addition to these indicators, tumor molecular features are now being incorporated into survival models for GBM subjects. Well-characterized molecular alterations include isocitrate dehydrogenase (IDH) mutation, 1p and 19q codeletion, epidermal growth factor receptor variant III (EGFRvIII) rearrangement, and MGMT promoter methylation (**Table 1**). Point mutations in isocitrate dehydrogenase (IDH) 1 and 2 have been associated with improved prognosis compared to patients with wild-type IDH [10]. The combined loss of chromosomal arms 1p and 19q has been shown to occur in

http://dx.doi.org/10.5772/64611

Molecular marker	Description	Prognostic role
IDH mutation	Increases production of 2-hydroxyglutarate also IDH1 mutation associated with CpG island methylator phenotype in gliomas	Favorable
1p/19q co-deletion	Currently unclear	Favorable, better treatment response to chemotherapy and radiation therapy
EGFRvIII	Ligand-independent receptor activation leading to increased proliferation and reduced apoptosis	Reduced long-term survival
MGMT hypermethylation	Reduced DNA repair	MGMT promoter methylation associated with prolonged progression-free and overall survival with treatment of alkylating chemotherapeutic agents

Table 1. Molecular prognostic factors associated with gliomas.

oligodendrogliomas and oligoastrocytomas [11], but it is associated with better response to chemotherapy and radiation therapy leading to prolonged progression-free and overall survival [12, 13]. Epidermal growth factor receptor (EGFR) is a cell surface receptor involved in cell proliferation. A common alteration of EGFR is a truncated version called EGFRvIII, which is constitutively active leading to increased cell proliferation and reduced apoptosis [14]. Overexpression of EGFRvIII is observed in 24–67% of GBM [15]. Since EGFRvIII is a unique surface receptor, strategies to target this epitope have been explored; additional details will be discussed in the tumor vaccine section. Finally, O^6-methylguanine methyltransferase (MGMT) is involved in the DNA repair pathway. Therefore, promoter methylation will lead to decreased protein levels and inability to repair the DNA. As such, promotor hypermethylation of MGMT has been observed in 20–40% of GBM [16]. The results from clinical trials and cohort studies have demonstrated that MGMT promoter methylation status is associated with prolonged progression-free and overall survival in patients with GBM treated with an alkylating chemotherapeutic agent [17–19].

3. Standard treatment regimen

The approach to GBM treatment has largely remained unchanged since 2005 with the publication of the Stupp et al. [20]. In this study, Stupp et al. [20] showed that giving temozolomide (TMZ) concurrently with radiation therapy after debulking surgery and then again following radiation therapy improved median survival in patients with newly diagnosed GBM. Each component of the Stupp protocol is important in the management of GBM. Surgery plays an important role as it allows for cytoreduction and histological confirmation of diagnosis. Achieving a gross total resection of >98% results in median survival of 12–15 months survival [21]. Approaches have been developed to aid surgeons in achieving a gross total resection while preserving baseline cognitive function. These include intraoperative MRI and neuronavigation, use of fluoride dye and imaging, and use of intraoperative brain mapping. Advances in imaging technology have allowed surgeons to incorporate functional MRI (fMRI) and Diffusion tensor imaging (DTI) images into neuronavigation systems in order to improve achieving maximum safe resection [22]. Radiation therapy is also important in treating GBM with an improvement in medial survival from 3–4 months to 9–12 months [20, 23]. Finally, as mentioned previously, TMZ, an alkylating agent, has shown to improve median survival [20]. Several chemotherapeutic agents targeting different cellular pathways have been studied with various results, including inhibitors of epidermal growth factor receptor (EGFR), vascular endothelial growth factor (VEGFR), platelet-derived growth factor receptor (PDGFR), protein kinase C (PKC), mammalian target of rapamycin (mTOR), RAF-MEK-ERK pathway, and integrins [24]. Of note, an anti-VEGF monoclonal antibody, bevacizumab, which demonstrated improved progression-free survival in two randomized phase 3 clinical trials, failed to improve overall survival [25, 26]. Therefore, advancing the realm of neurochemotherapeutic agents hinges on our understanding of disease mechanism and may benefit from a combined multimodality approach utilizing various targets and approaches.

4. Immunotherapy

The concept of immunotherapy for cancer treatment is based on stimulating the body's own immune system, predominately cytotoxic T lymphocytes (CTL), to target and eliminate tumor cells. This concept is based on the body's own defense mechanism to eliminate cells that have undergone malignant transformation in a process called immune surveillance [27]. Theoretically, if the host immune system is stimulated with expansion of sufficient numbers of tumor-specific CTLs or non-functioning T cells are rescued within the tumor microenvironment, cell-mediated lysis of tumor cells could lead to tumor regression [28]. These concepts have been applied to several non-CNS malignancies with promising results [29]. However, because the CNS was originally considered to be an immune-privileged site, immunotherapy approaches for CNS malignancies were deemed futile. The notion of the CNS being immune-privileged stems from studies in which rat osteosarcoma cells injected intracranially grew significantly better than cells injected subcutaneously or intramuscularly [30]. Additional evidence has historically been that since there is an intact blood brain barrier (BBB), the CNS and specifically the brain are presumed to be immune privileged.

Despite this antiquated line of thinking, more recent observations indicate that the CNS is actually immunospecialized. This is based on the considerable interaction observed with the peripheral nervous system and the non-parenchymal ventricles, meninges, and subarachnoid space [31]. For example, antigen presenting cells (APCs) are found in many areas of the brain, including leptomeninges, ventricles, and perivascular spaces [32, 33]. Additionally, recent evidence has emerged indicating that the CNS possesses a functional lymphatic system, which is located within the walls of dural sinuses and actually communicates with deep cervical lymph nodes [34–36]. This network is able to transport immune cells and macromolecules and serves as a mechanism for antigens to pass through the walls of cerebral arteries and be carried to the cervical lymph nodes through the Virchow-Robin perivascular spaces [37]. Interestingly, dendritic cells (DC) have been shown to travel outside the brain and present antigens to T cells located in the cervical lymph nodes [38]. This presentation of CNS antigens primes T cells for homing and infiltration to the tumor parenchyma [30]. Inflammatory stimuli, such as those induced by brain tumors, also increase CNS immunogenicity by provoking microglial activation and blood-brain barrier (BBB) disruption [39]. BBB disruption occurs secondary to glioma cell invasion of the basement membrane. This disruption also enables immune cells to migrate past the BBB, which normally would be intact, preventing such migration. As our understanding of immune function expands in the CNS, the field of immunotherapy as it pertains to CNS disease has emerged as a frontier player in the fight for CNS cancer. As a result, there are several immunotherapies currently being investigated in clinical trials with many producing promising results [30].

4.1. Tumor vaccines

The idea behind tumor vaccinations is to present tumor-associated antigens (TAAs) to the host immune system in order to evoke a pro-inflammatory antitumor response elicited by $CD4^+$ and $CD8^+$ T cells interacting with major histocompatibility complexes (MHC) I and MHC II, respectively [40]. Naturally, the success of tumor vaccinations and elegance of using this approach are that it is both tumor specific and subject specific, thereby, reducing inadvertent toxic side effects [40, 41]. Although there is great specificity in using tumor vaccinations, the challenge remains in optimizing the selection of targeted peptides since many TAAs are identified as "self" by the immune system [42]. Tumor vaccinations can be categorized according to their delivery method and includes peptide, dendritic cells (DCs), and heat shock protein (HSP).

Although several TAAs specific to GBM have been described in the literature including HER-2, gp100 [43], MAGE-1 [43], ATIA [44], and AIM-2 [45], peptide vaccination development using epidermal growth factor receptor variant III (EGFRvIII) has received the most attention [43]. First described by Heimberger et al. in 2003, the EGFRvIII vaccine, rindopepimut has been studied in several clinical trials with promising results [30, 46]. In a multicenter phase II trial, subjects with EGFRvIII-expressing GBM that received rindopepimut had a median progression-free survival from time of histological diagnosis of 14.2 months and an overall survival of 26.0 months [47]. In another multicenter phase II clinical trial (ACT III), the median overall survival was 21.8 months, which further confirms the results from the aforementioned phase II trial [48].

While these results are encouraging, a recent phase III clinical trial (ACT IV) evaluating rindopepimut was discontinued on the recommendations of the independent Data Safety and Monitoring Board based on observations that the treatment arm and control arms of the study were performing on *par* with each other and unlikely to meet its primary overall survival endpoint [49]. Another issue complicating the use of tumor peptide vaccinations is the notion that tumor recurrence post-peptide vaccination leads to altered tumor protein expression, which makes treatment approaches for tumor recurrences more challenging. Specifically, Sampson et al. analyzed those patients who received rindopepimut and subsequently experienced a recurrence. They demonstrated that in those tumors that recurred, 82% demonstrated loss of EGFRvIII expression. These results suggest that the peptide vaccine is able to successfully target EGFRvIII-expressing tumor cells. At the same time, these results indicate that the peptide vaccine preferentially led to the selection of EGFRvIII-negative tumor cells, resulting in tumor regrowth [47]. Despite this obstacle, one proposed strategy to overcoming this tumor event is to target multiple TAAs in an attempt to overcome the inherent heterogeneity of GBMs [40].

Still another approach to generate tumor vaccines while addressing the limitations of using one antigen is the use of heat shock protein (HSP) peptide complexes. HSP vaccines are generated from TAAs bound to HSP peptide complexes derived from GBM tissue. Two HSP peptide complexes that are currently being evaluated in clinical trials include HSP 70 and 96 [30]. In a phase II clinical trial, which evaluated a HSP peptide complex 96 vaccine, the authors demonstrated an increase in median overall survival of 42.6 weeks compared to historical controls [50]. Other HSPs, including HSP47, have been found to play a role in GBM pathogenesis specifically glioma angiogenesis and may serve as additional therapeutic targets [51, 52].

Several dendritic cell (DC) vaccines are currently being evaluated in various stages of clinical trials [30]. The mechanism of action for the majority of dendritic cell vaccines involves extracting autologous DC from the subject. Then *in vitro*, the DCs are stimulated or pulsed with tumor peptides or tumor lysate and subsequently re-introduced into the subject. The results of a phase I trial demonstrated a median progression-free survival of 16.9 months and median overall survival of 38.4 months after administration of a multi-epitope-pulsed DC vaccine [53]. In another phase I trial, median overall survival was 31.4 months after treatment with pulsed DCs followed by adjuvant treatment with either imiquimod or poly-ICLC [54]. In the latter study, the authors observed that subjects with GBMs with a mesenchymal gene expression profile were more susceptible to the DC treatment approach [54]. This observation underscores the importance of molecular characterization and developing a personal treatment approach.

Interestingly, as technologies advance, we now have the capability to develop computational modeling to identify potential tumor antigens through next-generation sequencing to identify mutations and peptide affinity algorithms to find peptides with high peptide-MHC affinity [30, 55, 56]. This approach has been validated in preclinical studies using melanoma cell lines [55]. It is currently unclear whether this approach can have similar efficacy against CNS tumors.

4.2. Immune checkpoint molecules

Many clinical studies are focusing on how to rescue the function of immune cells against non-immunogenic tumors and their immune suppressive microenvironments. It is well established that inhibitory receptors on T cells play a vital role in suppressing T cell-mediated antitumor responses [30, 57]. These inhibitory receptors, referred to as immune checkpoints, serve to prevent inappropriate or prolonged activation of the host immune system. There are several immune checkpoint protein inhibitors that have been developed and are demonstrating promising antitumor responses clinically—CTLA-4 and PD-L1 [30]. CTLA-4 has been shown to modulate T cell activation, thereby preventing unabated activation and proliferation [58]. A humanized CTLA-4 antibody, ipilimumab, has been FDA-approved and shown to have promising results in treating metastatic melanoma with an approximately 10.9% overall response rate that remains durable [59]. In the setting of GBM, administration of ipilimumab has been limited to small cohorts [30]. PD-LI is modulated by the PI(3)K-Akt-mTOR pathway [60] and its function is to suppress the proliferation and function of CTLs and also promote regulatory T cells (Tregs) activity through the binding of programmed cell death—1 (PD-1) [61]. PD-L1 is also found on the surface of GBM tumor cells, and expression is correlated with tumor grade and prognosis [62, 63].

Not surprisingly, the most promising outcomes regarding immune checkpoint therapy have been achieved through dual CTLA-4 and PD-L1 blockade. In a recent randomized controlled trial, blocking both CTLA-4 and PD-L1 in patients with advanced untreated melanoma resulted in a median progression-free survival of 11.5 months compared to CTLA-4 monotherapy with 2.9 months and PD-L1 monotherapy with 6.9 months [64]. Additionally, other checkpoint molecules (*e.g.*, LAG-3 and TIM-3) are currently being investigated in combination with PD-1 blockage in preclinical studies treating non-CNS tumors [65, 66]. With success in non-CNS tumor models, this strategy may also be effective in treating GBM and other CNS malignancies.

4.3. Human cytomegalovirus

Human cytomegalovirus (HCMV) was first reported to be associated with GBM in 2002 by Cobbs et al. [67]. Since that time, there has been much controversy surround this topic with a high degree of variability in the literature regarding the detection of HCMV in CNS tumors [67–92]. To help resolve some of this controversy, a consensus paper was published in 2012 [93]. Despite this, a consensus paper stating the existence of HCMV in gliomas and their potential role in tumorigenesis, recent studies using next-generation sequencing have not been able to identify any HCMV in CNS tumor tissue [73, 81, 85–87, 92, 93]. Furthermore, anti-CMV therapy has been relatively unremarkable in the clinical setting with results being unclear and several clinical trials currently underway. For example, results from the Sweden (VIGAS) study, a randomized, double-blinded, placebo-controlled trial published in 2013, demonstrated trends but no significant differences in tumor volumes between the valganciclovir (an anti-CMV drug) and placebo groups at 3 and 6 months [94]. However, when the authors performed a retrospective analysis of the same cohort adding in additional patients taking valganciclovir for compassionate reasons, the rate of survival of treated patients at 2 years was 62%, as compared with 18% of contemporary matched controls [95]. The conclusion as to whether HCMV is associated with GBM remains unclear and warrants additional studies to completely resolve this ongoing issue.

5. Advancing treatment products

In a concerted effort to combat CNS malignancies, the Brain Tumor Biotech Summit was created as a way to bring the private sector and researchers together to discuss and exchange novel ideas that would ultimately lead to advances in CNS malignancy therapy [96]. From this summit, several products were highlighted, all of which demonstrate promising results. ONC201/TIC10 is a small molecule drug that can cross the BBB [97] and effectively target the tumor necrosis factor-related apoptosis-inducing ligand (TRAIL) pathway in both cancer stem cells and tumor cells [96]. Preclinical studies in GBM and colorectal tumors have shown promising results with regression of tumors without adverse side effects [98, 99]. Several vaccines are currently being developed including the Prophage Series G-100 and G-200 vaccines, which utilize the HSP complex 96 purified from tumor tissue [96], synthetic immune-stimulant multi-peptide SL-701 DC vaccine [96], and EGFRvIII vaccine [47, 48, 100, 101]. SL-701 is derived from several unregulated factors in GBM, including IL-13Ralpha2, EphA2, and surviving [96].

ANG1005 is an angiopep-2-paclitaxel chemotherapeutic agent conjugated to cellular receptor ligand, LRP-1 [102, 103]. LRP-1 is highly expressed on the surface of the BBB and allows for entry into the brain parenchyma since LRP-1 is also highly expressed in GBM [103, 104]. Another cellular receptor ligand being investigated is HER2 receptor, which may be useful in targeting breast cancer brain metastases since HER2 receptor has been shown to be overexpressed in roughly 25–30% of breast cancers [105, 106]. Toca 511 is a replicating amphotropic murine leukemia virus that preferentially infects malignant cells and delivers cytosine deaminase (CD) protein. Inside malignant cells, the CD enzyme converts the antifungal drug 5-FC (5-fluorocytosine) to the anticancer drug 5-FU (5-fluorouracil) [107]. A new form of brachytherapy seed has also been developed, ^{131}Cs, which has a higher mean energy and a shorter half-life, allowing for fewer radioactive seeds and reduced exposure to family members and medical staff [108].

The most recent FDA-approved treatment for GBM is Novocure's Optune device, which uses a noninvasive tumor treating field generator that results in the slowing and ultimate reversal of tumor growth [109, 110]. The concept of the device is that it creates low intensity, alternating electric fields within the tumor site that act on the electrically charged cellular components, thereby preventing normal cellular functions such as mitosis, which ultimately leads to tumor cell death [109]. In a prospective, randomized, multi-institutional control trial designed to compare the effectiveness and safety of newly diagnosed GBM subjects treated with Optune in combination with temozolomide (TMZ) (n = 210) to those treated with TMZ alone (n = 105), progression-free survival in the treatment arm was 7.1 months compared to 4.0 months in the TMZ only group [111]. In addition, overall survival was 20.5 months in the Optune and TMZ group compared to 15.6 months in the TMZ only group [111]. The median follow-up for the study was 38 months (range 18–60 months) [111]. The authors concluded that adding Optune to maintenance TMZ can significantly prolong progression-free and overall survival in patients with newly diagnosed GBM [111].

6. Conclusion

GBM is a highly heterogeneous disease requiring a meticulous treatment approach. Despite advances in treatment options over the past decades, overall survival has remained relatively unchanged. As our understanding of GBM tumorigenesis increases, our treatment efforts have become more targeted. With tremendous strides in immunotherapy and biotechnology, the field of neurooncology holds promise for improving survival in those patients with CNS cancer. The notion of highly specific therapy with minimal side effects is

http://dx.doi.org/10.5772/64611

the benchmark for all cancer therapies striving to accomplish. As we usher in this new era in treating CNS tumors, our approach to fighting CNS disease will change with the ultimate goal of improved survivorship.

Author details

Michael J. Strong[1,2] and Marcus L. Ware[2,3*]

*Address all correspondence to: mware@ochsner.org

1 Department of Pathology, Tulane University School of Medicine, New Orleans, LA, USA

2 Department of Neurological Surgery, Ochsner Clinic Foundation, New Orleans, LA, USA

3 The University of Queensland School of Medicine, Ochsner Clinical School, New Orleans, LA, USA

References

[1] Ostrom QT, Gittleman H, Fulop J, Liu M, Blanda R, et al. CBTRUS statistical report: primary brain and central nervous system tumors diagnosed in the United States in 2008-2012. Neuro-oncology. 2015;17(suppl 4):iv1–iv62.

[2] Wen PY, Kesari S. Malignant gliomas in adults. New England Journal of Medicine. 2008;359(5):492–507.

[3] Ohgaki H, Kleihues P. Population-based studies on incidence, survival rates, and genetic alterations in astrocytic and oligodendroglial gliomas. Journal of Neuropathology and Experimental Neurology. 2005;64(6):479–89.

[4] Society AC. Cancer facts and figures 2015. Atlanta: American Cancer Society. 2015.

[5] Chandana S, Movva S, Arora M, Singh T. Primary brain tumors in adults. American Family Physician. 2008;77(10):1423–30.

[6] Verhaak RGW, Hoadley KA, Purdom E, Wang V, Qi Y, et al. Integrated genomic analysis identifies clinically relevant subtypes of glioblastoma characterized by abnormalities in PDGFRA, IDH1, EGFR, and NF1. Cancer Cell. 2010;17(1):98–110.

[7] Forsyth PA, Posner JB. Headaches in patients with brain tumors: a study of 111 patients. Neurology. 1993;43(9):1678–83.

[8] DeAngelis LM. Brain tumors. New England Journal of Medicine. 2001;344(2):114–23.

[9] Liigant A, Haldre S, Oun A, Linnamagi U, Saar A, et al. Seizure disorders in patients with brain tumors. European Neurology. 2001;45(1):46–51.

[10] Cohen A, Holmen S, Colman H. IDH1 and IDH2 mutations in gliomas. Current Neurology and Neuroscience Reports. 2013;13(5):1–7.

[11] Mur P, Mollejo M, Ruano Y, de Lope Á, Fiaño C, et al. Codeletion of 1p and 19q determines distinct gene methylation and expression profiles in IDH-mutated oligodendroglial tumors. Acta Neuropathologica. 2013;126(2):277–89.

[12] Cairncross G, Berkey B, Shaw E, Jenkins R, Scheithauer B, et al. Phase III trial of chemotherapy plus radiotherapy compared with radiotherapy alone for pure and mixed anaplastic oligodendroglioma: intergroup radiation therapy oncology group trial 9402. Journal of Clinical Oncology. 2006;24(18):2707–14.

[13] van den Bent M, Carpentier A, Brandes A, Sanson M, Taphoorn M, et al. Adjuvant procarbazine, lomustine, and vincristine improves progression-free survival but not overall survival in newly diagnosed anaplastic oligodendrogliomas and oligoastrocytomas: a randomized European Organisation for Research and Treatment of Cancer phase III trial. Journal of Clinical Oncology. 2006;24(18):2715–22.

[14] Batra S, Castelino-Prabhu S, Wikstrand C, Zhu X, Humphrey P, et al. Epidermal growth factor ligand-independent, unregulated, cell-transforming potential of a naturally occurring human mutant EGFRvIII gene. Cell Growth and Differentiation. 1995;6(10):1251–59.

[15] Heimberger AB, Suki D, Yang D, Shi W, Aldape K. The natural history of EGFR and EGFRvIII in glioblastoma patients. Journal of Translational Medicine. 2005;3:38.

[16] Ostrom Q, Cohen ML, Ondracek A, Sloan A, Barnholtz-Sloan J. Gene markers in brain tumors: what the epileptologist should know. Epilepsia. 2013;54:25–29.

[17] Esteller M, Garcia-Foncillas J, Andion E, Goodman SN, Hidalgo OF, et al. Inactivation of the DNA-repair gene MGMT and the clinical response of gliomas to alkylating agents. New England Journal of Medicine. 2000;343(19):1350–54.

[18] Hegi ME, Diserens A-C, Godard S, Dietrich P-Y, Regli L, et al. Clinical trial substantiates the predictive value of *O*-6-methylguanine-DNA methyltransferase promoter methylation in glioblastoma patients treated with temozolomide. Clinical Cancer Research. 2004;10(6):1871–74.

[19] Hegi ME, Diserens A-C, Gorlia T, Hamou M-F, de Tribolet N, et al. MGMT gene silencing and benefit from temozolomide in glioblastoma. New England Journal of Medicine. 2005;352(10):997–1003.

[20] Stupp R, Mason WP, van den Bent MJ, Weller M, Fisher B, et al. Radiotherapy plus concomitant and adjuvant temozolomide for glioblastoma. New England Journal of Medicine. 2005;352(10):987–96.

[21] Hentschel SJ, Sawaya R. Optimizing outcomes with maximal surgical resection of malignant gliomas. Cancer Control. 2003;10(2):109–14.

[22] Rasmussen IA, Jr., Lindseth F, Rygh OM, Berntsen EM, Selbekk T, et al. Functional neuronavigation combined with intra-operative 3D ultrasound: initial experiences during surgical resections close to eloquent brain areas and future directions in automatic brain shift compensation of preoperative data. Acta Neurochirurgica. 2007;149(4):365–78.

[23] Walker MD, Alexander E, Hunt WE, MacCarty CS, Mahaley MS, et al. Evaluation of BCNU and/or radiotherapy in the treatment of anaplastic gliomas. Journal of Neurosurgery. 1978;49(3):333–43.

[24] Minniti G, Muni R, Lanzetta G, Marchetti P, Enrici RM. Chemotherapy for glioblastoma: current treatment and future perspectives for cytotoxic and targeted agents. Anticancer Research. 2009;29(12):5171–84.

[25] Gilbert MR, Dignam JJ, Armstrong TS, Wefel JS, Blumenthal DT, et al. A randomized trial of bevacizumab for newly diagnosed glioblastoma. New England Journal of Medicine. 2014;370(8):699–708.

[26] Chinot OL, Wick W, Mason W, Henriksson R, Saran F, et al. Bevacizumab plus radiotherapy–temozolomide for newly diagnosed glioblastoma. New England Journal of Medicine. 2014;370(8):709–22.

[27] Vesely MD, Kershaw MH, Schreiber RD, Smyth MJ. Natural innate and adaptive immunity to cancer. Annual Review of Immunology. 2011;29(1):235–71.

[28] Kronik N, Kogan Y, Elishmereni M, Halevi-Tobias K, Vuk-Pavlović S, et al. Predicting outcomes of prostate cancer immunotherapy by personalized mathematical models. PLoS One. 2010;5(12):e15482.

[29] Khalil DN, Smith EL, Brentjens RJ, Wolchok JD. The future of cancer treatment: immunomodulation, CARs and combination immunotherapy. Nature Reviews Clinical Oncology. 2016;13(5):273–90.

[30] Binder DC, Davis AA, Wainwright DA. Immunotherapy for cancer in the central nervous system: current and future directions. Oncoimmunology. 2016;5(2):e1082027.

[31] Carson MJ, Doose JM, Melchior B, Schmid CD, Ploix CC. CNS immune privilege: hiding in plain sight. Immunological Reviews. 2006;213(1):48–65.

[32] D'Agostino PM, Gottfried-Blackmore A, Anandasabapathy N, Bulloch K. Brain dendritic cells: biology and pathology. Acta Neuropathologica. 2012;124(5):599–614.

[33] Bechmann I, Galea I, Perry VH. What is the blood-brain barrier (not)? Trends in Immunology. 2007;28(1):5–11.

[34] Louveau A, Harris TH, Kipnis J. Revisiting the mechanisms of CNS immune privilege. Trends in Immunology. 2015;36(10):569–77.

[35] Louveau A, Smirnov I, Keyes TJ, Eccles JD, Rouhani SJ, et al. Structural and functional features of central nervous system lymphatic vessels. Nature. 2015;523(7560):337–41.

[36] Aspelund A, Antila S, Proulx ST, Karlsen TV, Karaman S, et al. A dural lymphatic vascular system that drains brain interstitial fluid and macromolecules. The Journal of Experimental Medicine. 2015;212(7):991–99.

[37] Cserr HF, Harling-Berg CJ, Knopf PM. Drainage of brain extracellular fluid into blood and deep cervical lymph and its immunological significance. Brain Pathology. 1992;2(4):269–76.

[38] Mohammad MG, Tsai VWW, Ruitenberg MJ, Hassanpour M, Li H, et al. Immune cell trafficking from the brain maintains CNS immune tolerance. The Journal of Clinical Investigation. 2014;124(3):1228–41.

[39] Rivest S. Regulation of innate immune responses in the brain. Nature Reviews Immunology. 2009;9(6):429–39.

[40] Oh T, Sayegh ET, Fakurnejad S, Oyon D, Lamano JB, et al. Vaccine therapies in malignant glioma. Current Neurology and Neuroscience Reports. 2014;15(1):1–7.

[41] Tanaka S, Louis DN, Curry WT, Batchelor TT, Dietrich J. Diagnostic and therapeutic avenues for glioblastoma: no longer a dead end? Nature Clinical Practice Oncology. 2013;10(1):14–26.

[42] Schietinger A, Philip M, Schreiber H. Specificity in cancer immunotherapy. Seminars in Immunology. 2008;20(5):276–85.

[43] Liu G, Ying H, Zeng G, Wheeler CJ, Black KL, et al. HER-2, gp100, and MAGE-1 are expressed in human glioblastoma and recognized by cytotoxic t cells. Cancer Research. 2004;64(14):4980.

[44] Choksi S, Lin Y, Pobezinskaya Y, Chen L, Park C, et al. A HIF-1 Target, ATIA, protects cells from apoptosis by modulating the mitochondrial thioredoxin, TRX2. Molecular Cell. 2011;42(5):597–609.

[45] Liu G, Yu JS, Zeng G, Yin D, Xie D, et al. AIM-2: a novel tumor antigen is expressed and presented by human glioma cells. Journal of Immunotherapy. 2004;27(3):220–26.

[46] Heimberger AB, Crotty LE, Archer GE, Hess KR, Wikstrand CJ, et al. Epidermal growth factor receptor VIII peptide vaccination is efficacious against established intracerebral tumors. Clinical Cancer Research. 2003;9(11):4247.

[47] Sampson JH, Heimberger AB, Archer GE, Aldape KD, Friedman AH, et al. Immunologic escape after prolonged progression-free survival with epidermal growth factor receptor variant iii peptide vaccination in patients with newly diagnosed glioblastoma. Journal of Clinical Oncology. 2010;28(31):4722–29.

[48] Schuster J, Lai RK, Recht LD, Reardon DA, Paleologos NA, et al. A phase II, multicenter trial of rindopepimut (CDX-110) in newly diagnosed glioblastoma: the ACT III study. Neuro-oncology. 2015;17(6):854–61.

[49] Celldex. The Phase 3 ACT IV Study of RINTEGA in newly diagnosed glioblastoma (discontinued) 2016 [August 28, 2016]. Available from: http://www.celldex.com/pipeline/rindopepimut.php.

[50] Bloch O, Crane CA, Fuks Y, Kaur R, Aghi MK, et al. Heat-shock protein peptide complex–96 vaccination for recurrent glioblastoma: a phase II, single-arm trial. Neuro-oncology. 2014;16(2):274–79.

[51] Wu ZB, Cai L, Lin SJ, Leng ZG, Guo YH, et al. Heat shock protein 47 promotes glioma angiogenesis. Brain Pathology. 2016;26(1):31–42.

[52] Wu ZB, Cai L, Qiu C, Zhang AL, Lin SJ, et al. CTL responses to HSP47 associated with the prolonged survival of patients with glioblastomas. Neurology. 2014;82(14):1261–65.

[53] Phuphanich S, Wheeler CJ, Rudnick JD, Mazer M, Wang H, et al. Phase I trial of a multi-epitope-pulsed dendritic cell vaccine for patients with newly diagnosed glioblastoma. Cancer Immunology, Immunotherapy. 2013;62(1):125–35.

[54] Prins RM, Soto H, Konkankit V, Odesa SK, Eskin A, et al. Gene expression profile correlates with t-cell infiltration and relative survival in glioblastoma patients vaccinated with dendritic cell immunotherapy. Clinical Cancer Research. 2011;17(6):1603.

[55] Robbins PF, Lu Y-C, El-Gamil M, Li YF, Gross C, et al. Mining exomic sequencing data to identify mutated antigens recognized by adoptively transferred tumor-reactive T cells. Nature Medicine. 2013;19(6):747–52.

[56] Binder DC, Schreiber H. High-affinity peptide-based anticancer vaccination to overcome resistance to immunostimulatory antibodies. Oncoimmunology. 2013;2(12):e26704.

[57] Leach DR, Krummel MF, Allison JP. Enhancement of antitumor immunity by CTLA-4 blockade. Science. 1996;271(5256):1734.

[58] Scheipers P, Reiser H. Role of the CTLA-4 receptor in t cell activation and immunity. Immunologic Research. 1998;18(2):103–15.

[59] Hodi FS, O'Day SJ, McDermott DF, Weber RW, Sosman JA, et al. Improved survival with Ipilimumab in patients with metastatic melanoma. New England Journal of Medicine. 2010;363(8):711–23.

[60] Parsa AT, Waldron JS, Panner A, Crane CA, Parney IF, et al. Loss of tumor suppressor PTEN function increases B7-H1 expression and immunoresistance in glioma. Nature Medicine. 2007;13(1):84–88.

[61] Lipson EJ, Forde PM, Hammers H-J, Emens LA, Taube JM, et al. Antagonists of PD-1 and PD-L1 in cancer treatment. Seminars in Oncology. 2015;42(4):587–600.

[62] Wilmotte R, Burkhardt K, Kindler V, Belkouch M-C, Dussex G, et al. B7-homolog 1 expression by human glioma: a new mechanism of immune evasion. NeuroReport. 2005;16(10):1081–85.

[63] Wei B, Wang L, Zhao X, Du C, Guo Y, et al. The upregulation of programmed death 1 on peripheral blood T cells of glioma is correlated with disease progression. Tumor Biology. 2014;35(4):2923–29.

[64] Larkin J, Chiarion-Sileni V, Gonzalez R, Grob JJ, Cowey CL, et al. Combined nivolumab and ipilimumab or monotherapy in untreated melanoma. New England Journal of Medicine. 2015;373(1):23–34.

[65] Woo S-R, Turnis ME, Goldberg MV, Bankoti J, Selby M, et al. Immune inhibitory molecules LAG-3 and PD-1 synergistically regulate T-cell function to promote tumoral immune escape. Cancer Research. 2012;72(4):917.

[66] Sakuishi K, Apetoh L, Sullivan JM, Blazar BR, Kuchroo VK, et al. Targeting Tim-3 and PD-1 pathways to reverse T cell exhaustion and restore anti-tumor immunity. The Journal of Experimental Medicine. 2010;207(10):2187–94.

[67] Cobbs CS, Harkins L, Samanta M, Gillespie GY, Bharara S, et al. Human cytomegalovirus infection and expression in human malignant glioma. Cancer Research. 2002;62(12):3347–50.

[68] Lau SK, Chen Y-Y, Chen W-G, Diamond DJ, Mamelak AN, et al. Lack of association of cytomegalovirus with human brain tumors. Modern Pathology. 2005;18(6):838–43.

[69] Mitchell DA, Xie W, Schmittling R, Learn C, Friedman A, et al. Sensitive detection of human cytomegalovirus in tumors and peripheral blood of patients diagnosed with glioblastoma. Neuro-oncology. 2008;10(1):10–18.

[70] Poltermann S, Schlehofer B, Steindorf K, Schnitzler P, Geletneky K, et al. Lack of association of herpesviruses with brain tumors. Journal of Neurovirology. 2006;12(2):90–99.

[71] Saddawi-Konefka R, Crawford J. Chronic viral infection and primary central nervous system malignancy. Journal of Neuroimmune Pharmacology. 2010;5(3):387–403.

[72] Scheurer M, Bondy M, Aldape K, Albrecht T, El-Zein R. Detection of human cytomegalovirus in different histological types of gliomas. Acta Neuropathologica. 2008;116(1):79–86.

[73] Tang K-W, Alaei-Mahabadi B, Samuelsson T, Lindh M, Larsson E. The landscape of viral expression and host gene fusion and adaptation in human cancer. Nature Communications. 2013; 4: 2513.

[74] Sabatier J, Uro-Coste E, Pommepuy I, Labrousse F, Allart S, et al. Detection of human cytomegalovirus genome and gene products in central nervous system tumours. British Journal of Cancer. 2005;92(4):747–50.

[75] Slinger E, Maussang D, Schreiber A, Siderius M, Rahbar A, et al. HCMV-encoded chemokine receptor US28 mediates proliferative signaling through the IL-6–STAT3 axis. Science Signaling. 2010;3(133):ra58.

[76] Lucas K, Bao L, Bruggeman R, Dunham K, Specht C. The detection of CMV pp65 and IE1 in glioblastoma multiforme. Journal of Neurooncology. 2011;103(2):231–38.

[77] Ranganathan P, Clark PA, Kuo JS, Salamat MS, Kalejta RF. Significant association of multiple human cytomegalovirus genomic loci with glioblastoma multiforme samples. Journal of Virology. 2012;86(2):854–64.

[78] Rahbar A, Stragliotto G, Orrego A, Peredo I, Taher C, et al. Low levels of human cytomegalovirus infection in glioblastoma multiforme associates with patient survival; -a case-control study. Herpesviridae. 2012;3(1):3.

[79] Bhattacharjee B, Renzette N, Kowalik TF. Genetic analysis of cytomegalovirus in malignant gliomas. Journal of Virology. 2012;86(12):6815–24.

[80] Fonseca RF, Kawamura MT, Oliveira JA, Teixeira A, Alves G, et al. The prevalence of human cytomegalovirus DNA in gliomas of Brazilian patients. Memórias do Instituto Oswaldo Cruz. 2012;107:953–54.

[81] Khoury JD, Tannir NM, Williams MD, Chen Y, Yao H, et al. Landscape of DNA virus associations across human malignant cancers: analysis of 3,775 cases using RNA-Seq. Journal of Virology. 2013;87(16):8916–26.

[82] Rahbar A, Orrego A, Peredo I, Dzabic M, Wolmer-Solberg N, et al. Human cytomegalovirus infection levels in glioblastoma multiforme are of prognostic value for survival. Journal of Clinical Virology. 2013;57(1):36–42.

[83] Ding D, Han S, Wang Z, Guo Z, Wu A. Does the existence of HCMV components predict poor prognosis in glioma? Journal of Neurooncology. 2014;116(3):515–22.

[84] dos Santos CJ, Stangherlin LM, Figueiredo EG, Corrêa C, Teixeira MJ, et al. High prevalence of HCMV and viral load in tumor tissues and peripheral blood of glioblastoma multiforme patients. Journal of Medical Virology. 2014;86(11):1953–61.

[85] Tang K-W, Hellstrand K, Larsson E. Absence of cytomegalovirus in high-coverage DNA sequencing of human glioblastoma multiforme. International Journal of Cancer. 2015;136(4):977–81.

[86] Cimino PJ, Zhao G, Wang D, Sehn JK, Lewis Jr JS, et al. Detection of viral pathogens in high grade gliomas from unmapped next-generation sequencing data. Experimental and Molecular Pathology. 2014;96(3):310–15.

[87] Cosset É, Petty TJ, Dutoit V, Cordey S, Padioleau I, et al. Comprehensive metagenomic analysis of glioblastoma reveals absence of known virus despite antiviral-like type I interferon gene response. International Journal of Cancer. 2014;135(6):1381–89.

[88] Yamashita Y, Ito Y, Isomura H, Takemura N, Okamoto A, et al. Lack of presence of the human cytomegalovirus in human glioblastoma. Modern Pathology. 2014;27(7):922–29.

[89] Bianchi E, Roncarati P, Hougrand O, Guérin-El Khourouj V, Boreux R, et al. Human cytomegalovirus and primary intracranial tumors: frequency of tumor infection and lack of correlation with systemic immune anti-viral responses. Neuropathology and Applied Neurobiology. 2015; 41(2): e29-40.

[90] Baumgarten P, Michaelis M, Rothweiler F, Starzetz T, Rabenau HF, et al. Human cytomegalovirus infection in tumor cells of the nervous system is not detectable with standardized pathologico-virological diagnostics. Neuro-oncology. 2014;16(11):1469–77.

[91] Amirian ES, Bondy ML, Mo Q, Bainbridge MN, Scheurer ME. Presence of viral DNA in whole-genome sequencing of brain tumor tissues from the cancer genome atlas. Journal of Virology. 2014;88(1):774.

[92] Strong MJ, Blanchard E, Lin Z, Morris CA, Baddoo M, et al. A comprehensive next generation sequencing-based virome assessment in brain tissue suggests no major virus—tumor association. Acta Neuropathologica Communications. 2016;4(1):1–10.

[93] Dziurzynski K, Chang SM, Heimberger AB, Kalejta RF, McGregor Dallas SR, et al. Consensus on the role of human cytomegalovirus in glioblastoma. Neuro-oncology. 2012;14(3):246–55.

[94] Stragliotto G, Rahbar A, Solberg NW, Lilja A, Taher C, et al. Effects of valganciclovir as an add-on therapy in patients with cytomegalovirus-positive glioblastoma: a randomized, double-blind, hypothesis-generating study. International Journal of Cancer. 2013;133(5):1204–13.

[95] Soderberg-Naucler C, Rahbar A, Stragliotto G. Survival in patients with glioblastoma receiving valganciclovir. New England Journal of Medicine. 2013;369(10):985–86.

[96] Chakraborty S, Bodhinayake I, Chiluwal A, Langer DJ, Ruggieri R, et al. Neuro-oncology biotech industry progress report. Journal of Neurooncology. 2016;128(1):175–82.

[97] Greer YE, Lipkowitz S. TIC10/ONC201: a bend in the road to clinical development. Oncoscience. 2015;2(2):75–76.

[98] Prabhu VV, Allen JE, Dicker DT, El-Deiry WS. Small-molecule ONC201/TIC10 targets chemotherapy-resistant colorectal cancer stem–like cells in an Akt/Foxo3a/TRAIL–dependent manner. Cancer Research. 2015;75(7):1423.

[99] Karpel-Massler G, Bâ M, Shu C, Halatsch M-E, Westhoff M-A, et al. TIC10/ONC201 synergizes with Bcl-2/Bcl-xL inhibition in glioblastoma by suppression of Mcl-1 and its binding partners *in vitro* and *in vivo*. Oncotarget. 2015;6(34):36456–71.

[100] Babu R, Adamson DC. Rindopepimut: an evidence-based review of its therapeutic potential in the treatment of EGFRvIII-positive glioblastoma. Core Evidence. 2012;7:93–103.

[101] Sampson JH, Aldape KD, Archer GE, Coan A, Desjardins A, et al. Greater chemotherapy-induced lymphopenia enhances tumor-specific immune responses that eliminate EGFRvIII-expressing tumor cells in patients with glioblastoma. Neuro-oncology. 2011;13(3):324–33.

[102] Régina A, Demeule M, Ché C, Lavallée I, Poirier J, et al. Antitumour activity of ANG1005, a conjugate between paclitaxel and the new brain delivery vector Angiopep-2. British Journal of Pharmacology. 2008;155(2):185–97.

[103] Thomas FC, Taskar K, Rudraraju V, Goda S, Thorsheim HR, et al. Uptake of ANG1005, a novel paclitaxel derivative, through the blood-brain barrier into brain and experimental brain metastases of breast cancer. Pharmaceutical Research. 2009;26(11):2486–94.

[104] Bertrand Y, Currie JC, Poirier J, Demeule M, Abulrob A, et al. Influence of glioma tumour microenvironment on the transport of ANG1005 via low-density lipoprotein receptor-related protein 1. British Journal of Cancer. 2011;105(11):1697–707.

[105] Slamon DJ, Clark GM, Wong SG, Levin WJ, Ullrich A, et al. Human breast cancer: correlation of relapse and survival with amplification of the HER-2/neu oncogene. Science. 1987;235(4785):177.

[106] Slamon DJ, Godolphin W, Jones LA, Holt JA, Wong SG, et al. Studies of the HER-2/neu proto-oncogene in human breast and ovarian cancer. Science. 1989;244(4905):707.

[107] Nakamura H, Mullen JT, Chandrasekhar S, Pawlik TM, Yoon SS, et al. Multimodality therapy with a replication-conditional herpes simplex virus 1 mutant that expresses yeast cytosine deaminase for intratumoral conversion of 5-fluorocytosine to 5-fluorouracil. Cancer Research. 2001;61(14):5447.

[108] Wernicke AG, Yondorf MZ, Peng L, Trichter S, Nedialkova L, et al. Phase I/II study of resection and intraoperative cesium-131 radioisotope brachytherapy in patients with newly diagnosed brain metastases. Journal of Neurosurgery. 2014;121(2):338–48.

[109] Fonkem E, Wong ET. NovoTTF-100A: a new treatment modality for recurrent glioblastoma. Expert Review of Neurotherapeutics. 2012;12(8):895–99.

[110] Kirson ED, Dbalý V, Tovaryš F, Vymazal J, Soustiel JF, et al. Alternating electric fields arrest cell proliferation in animal tumor models and human brain tumors. Proceedings of the National Academy of Sciences. 2007;104(24):10152–57.

[111] Stupp R, Taillibert S, Kanner AA, Kesari S, Steinberg DM, et al. Maintenance therapy with tumor-treating fields plus temozolomide vs temozolomide alone for glioblastoma: a randomized clinical trial. Journal of the American Medical Association. 2015;314(23):2535–43.

Chapter 8

Primary Central Nervous System Lymphoma

Mihnea Zdrenghea, Delia Dima, Ciprian Tomuleasa,
Horia Bumbea and Cristina Bagacean

Additional information is available at the end of the chapter

http://dx.doi.org/10.5772/66601

Abstract

Although non-Hodgkin's lymphoma (NHL) is a frequent cancer worldwide, primary central nervous system (CNS) lymphoma (PCNSL) is a rare presentation, with an incidence of less than 0.5 per 100,000 persons-years in the western world. In the vast majority of cases, it has the histology of a diffuse large B-cell lymphoma (DLBCL) and is a hardly curable disease with high relapse risk. Therapeutic options are limited by blood-brain barrier penetration of drugs and because of its low-incidence high-grade evidence from large studies is lacking, current management being based on reports on rather small cohorts. The current standard first-line treatment for PCNSL consists of high-dose methotrexate (HD-MTX) in combination with a variety of drugs and consolidation whole-brain radiotherapy, the latter being progressively replaced by chemotherapy. For patients relapsing after first-line treatment, intensive chemotherapy with autologous stem cell support is a feasible and relatively safe salvage therapy. In the present chapter, we briefly discuss primary central nervous system lymphoma management and review current therapeutic options and evidence-based recommendations. We discuss the role of whole-brain radiotherapy (WBRT) and new prospects to avoid this side effect-ridden approach. Also, we will look at new therapeutic approaches currently under investigation, including immunotherapy.

Keywords: PCNSL, primary cerebral tumor, aggressive lymphoma, whole-brain radiotherapy, blood-brain barrier

1. Introduction

One of the deadliest hematologic malignancies of our days, primary central nervous system (CNS) lymphoma (PCNSL), is a major unmet in oncology, with an outcome similar to that of acute leukemia, and a commonly used phrase to coin this poor prognosis states that the majority of patients die of their disease.

Of all primary CNS tumors, PCNSL represents a small percentage of around 4% in the United States [1]. With the exception of rare, anecdotal reports of primary CNS Hodgkin's lymphoma, they are extranodal non-Hodgkin's lymphomas (NHLs), the vast majority being of aggressive, diffuse large B-cell type. According to the European Cancer Observatory's (EUCAN) national estimates report on cancer incidence in Europe, the mean EU 27 incidence in 2012 of brain and CNS tumors was of 6.9 per 100,000 persons, ranging from a high of 11.9 in Sweden to a low of 5 in Hungary, allowing for an estimate of around 0.3 new cases of PCNSL per 100,000 persons in 2012 across the EU.

The percentage of PCNSL presentation among all NHL cases is estimated at 2–3% [2]. More than 90% of PCNSL are diffuse large B-cell lymphomas (DLBCLs), other histological forms encountered being Burkitt's and lymphoblastic lymphomas (5%) and marginal zone and T-cell NHL (3%) [3]. These low-incidence figures underscore the difficulty in patient accrual for clinical studies and, implicitly, for the formulation of evidence-based recommendations. Therapeutic advance is thus difficult, in a tumor ranked as one of the deadliest lymphomas, with a present estimated cure rate lower than 50%. The 2016 World Health Organization classification update of lymphoid neoplasms lists primary DLBCL of the central nervous system as a distinct entity among mature lymphoid neoplasms [4].

The etiology of PCNSL is unknown, as with the majority of cancers. However, increased incidence is observed in HIV infection, PCNSL being, with 15–20% of all cases, one of the favorite presentations of AIDS-related lymphomas. The high incidence of PCNSL in AIDS patients declined with the advent of the contemporaneous highly active antiviral therapy, and an improvement in its prognosis was noted, as well [2]. An increased incidence is also observed in other immunosuppressed patients, notably in recipients of allogeneic transplantation on long-term immunosuppressive therapy. Although the spread of HIV infection offered a tempting explanation for the continuous increase in PCNSL (and NHL overall) incidence reported over the last decades of the twentieth century, the trend remains positive even after subtracting AIDS patients. As with many cancers, incidence of PCNSL increases with age, and it is estimated that approximately a half of the patients are over 65 years of age, with limiting implications in intensive management options. The disease favors men, with a 2:1 male to female gender ratio.

In the next sections, we will review the pathogenesis and diagnostic workup, as well as the current treatment paradigm for PCNSL. Novel therapeutic approaches currently under investigation will be also discussed

2. Pathobiology of PCNSL

Primary central nervous system lymphoma (PCNSL) has been historically known by many other names, including reticulum cell sarcoma, diffuse histiocytic lymphoma, and microglioma. The proliferation of names reflects initial uncertainty about the cell of origin. PCNSL is in the overwhelming majority of cases an aggressive extranodal diffuse B-cell lymphoma. The cell of origin of the tumor obviously belongs to the lymphoid lineage, but the lymphomatous histology of PCNSL was established only during the 1970s. Before that, PCNSL was regarded as a microglioma or reticulum cell sarcoma. The lack of a precise histological definition of the disease did not, however, impact on therapy outcomes in that era, as the sole therapeutic modality employed for brain tumors, besides surgery, was brain radiotherapy [5]. Evolution in the understanding of the pathobiology of PCNSL lagged behind that of nodal lymphomas because of the dame reasons that hampered therapeutic evolution, namely, the rarity of the tumor.

PCNSL is, in an overwhelming majority of approximately (95%) of cases, an aggressive extranodal diffuse large B-cell lymphoma (DLBCL) [6]. Other histologies have been described including lymphoma of T-cell origin, lymphoblastic lymphoma, Burkitt lymphoma, mucosa-associated lymphoid tissue (MALT), and marginal zone lymphoma (MZL) [7, 8]. Studies have generally focused on the features of primary DLBCL arising in the brain. Based on overexpression of B-cell lymphoma 6 (BCL-6) protein and V(H) gene sequence mutational status, PCNSL was thought to be of germinal center (GC) origin [9–11]. More recent immunohistochemical studies have shown that at least 95% of cases stain positive for MUM-1, regardless of their BCL-6 status; therefore, the majority have an activated B-cell (ABC) profile [12].The immunoprofile association with clinical outcome was evaluated, and high BCL-6 expression is usually associated with poor prognosis factors (elderly patients, high ECOG performance status) and correlates with refractory disease and shorter progression-free and overall survival [12, 13].

More recently, important progress has been made on the transcriptional profile of PCNSL. Overexpression of MYC, high expression of miRNA involved in MYC pathway, and MYC translocations have all been identified and seem to have an important role in this disease pathogenesis [13–15]. Other common genomic aberrations include loss of chromosome arm 6q and losses on 6p21 involving tumor suppressor genes, regulators of B-cell differentiation, and NF-κB signaling [16, 17]. In addition, activating mutations of CARD11 and MyD88 are recurrent in PCNSL and support the aberrant activation of NF-κB pathway [18, 19]. Given the distinct genomic features and the necessity of an adapted treatment, different from its systemic counterpart, PCNSL is now recognized as a distinct subtype of large B-cell lymphoma by the WHO [6, 20].

The selective tropism and whether PCNSL arises in the central nervous system (CNS) or outside the brain are still unresolved issues. The initial hypothesis was that B cells transform outside the CNS and due to certain adhesion molecules and chemokines, the modified lymphomatous cells have neurotropism and are preserved in the brain tissue [21]. Moreover, high chemokine CXCL-13 concentration in the cerebrospinal fluid (CSF) of PCNSL patients correlates with adverse prognosis and together with IL-10 are highly specific for the diagnosis of CNS lymphoma [22, 23].

The theory of development of neurotropic lymphomatous cells outside the brain was mainly based on the information that there is a lack of classical lymphatic drainage system in the CNS. A fundamental discovery that could change these assumptions about the pathogenesis of PCNSL was recently published and reports the presence of functional lymphatic vessels lining the dural sinuses, able to carry immune cells from the CSF to the deep cervical lymph nodes [24]. There is an ongoing controversy on the pathobiology of PCNSL, and new insights, which could change the current understanding of this disease group, are expected.

3. Clinical presentation, diagnosis and workup

The clinical presentation of PCNSL reflects its localization and typically consists of neurologic symptoms, which can be extremely polymorphic, depending on the tumor site. Psychiatric and ocular/visual manifestations are also common. Usually, these symptoms prompt neurologic imaging which points to the tumor. Despite significant progress in imaging techniques and in the interpretation, there is a significant risk in attributing too much diagnostic power to neuroimaging, succumbing to the temptation to formulate a diagnosis based on tumor appearance. Statistically, the most frequent localization of PCNSL is supratentorial and periventricular, accounting for approximately 80% of cases, and 60% of PCNSL are presenting as a single mass at diagnosis, but leptomeningeal, cerebellar, and intraocular presentations are not uncommon. CSF cytology is positive demonstrating meningeal involvement in 16% of cases, but only rarely (<5% of cases) is leptomeningeal disease present without a cerebral lesion. Primary spinal cord presentation is extremely rarely encountered [3]. Eye involvement is seen in up to 20% of patients, either as a primary localization or accompanying other CNS localizations. Also, subsequent development of brain lesions by spread from an initial intraocular localization is not uncommon [25]. Symptoms at presentation vary according to the tumor localization and may include headache, lethargy, visual disturbances, and focal neurological signs, while B symptoms are extremely uncommon [3].

The timely and correct diagnosis of primary CNS lymphoma can be significantly hampered by the administration of corticosteroid therapy, which occurs frequently in the neurological setting, where patients are likely to be referred because of their clinical presentation. Response to corticosteroid therapy has been and still is wrongly regarded as a major argument sustaining a lymphoma diagnosis in patients with brain tumors. Although corticosteroids are extremely active in lymphomas and can lead to a significant response and, sometimes, to the disappearance of the initial tumor, other histological types of primary CNS tumors may respond well to systemic corticosteroids, and thus response to corticosteroids cannot be regarded as an argument for the lymphomatous origin of the tumor. As with the vast majority of solid cancers, the correct positive diagnosis is anatomopathological (with rare exceptions discussed below) and involves the obtention of a bioptic fragment of the tumor. There is no evidence that surgical tumor removal is beneficial in lymphomas, and, thus, current evidence-based guidelines recommend a minimal invasive diagnostic approach for suspected CNS lymphoma, which is usually a stereotactic biopsy.

PCNSL workup consists of positive diagnosis and the evaluation of disease extension, patient status, prognostic markers, as well as treatment tolerance.

Clinical evaluation must include neurological examination, a general clinical exam, and performance status. Both ECOG/WHO score and Karnofsky performance status scale are used to assess status by different guidelines.

http://dx.doi.org/10.5772/66601

Imaging. In practice, it is not infrequent for a cerebral CT scan to be the first brain examination to describe the lymphoma, because of the typical patient presentation with neurological symptoms with a CT scan being employed to rule out ischemic or hemorrhagic stroke (**Figure 1**). Whole-brain MRI is the first step to sustain a suspicion of brain tumor, and it allows for the assessment of local extension of the brain tumor, as well as for the preparation of a minimal invasive bioptic approach for diagnosis. The MRI appearance can strongly suggest a lymphomatous nature of the tumor (**Figures 2–6**). **Figure 7** demonstrates the MRI appearance of a very good partial response after first-line chemoimmunotherapy, and **Figures 8–10** depict MRI appearance of a multifocal, bilateral relapse at 2 years. Complementary chest-abdominal-pelvic CT scan is the standard investigation for the exclusion of systemic disease, but PET-CT can replace it when available. Testicular examination including ultrasound may complete imaging, as testicular involvement is more frequent in cerebral lymphomas.

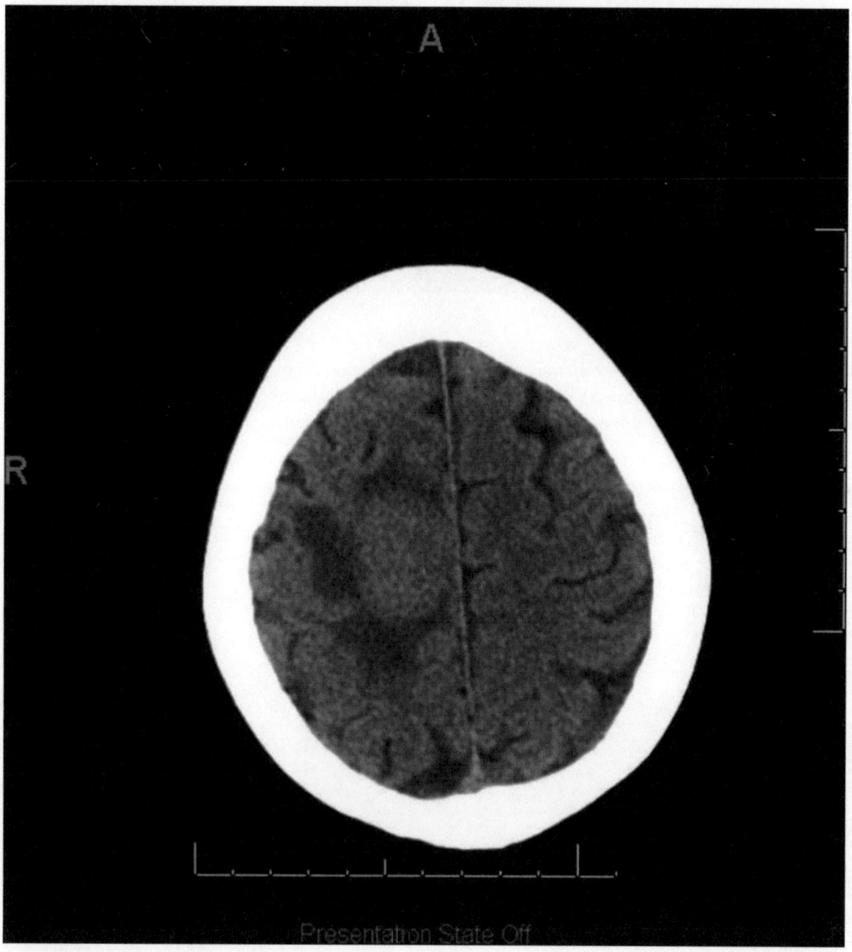

Figure 1. Nonenhanced CT of the head at presentation, axial slice at the level of the convexity, showing a single right subcortical frontoparietal mass. The lesion appears isodense to gray matter (suggestive for CNS lymphoma) surrounded by vasogenic edema. Please note gray matter sparing.

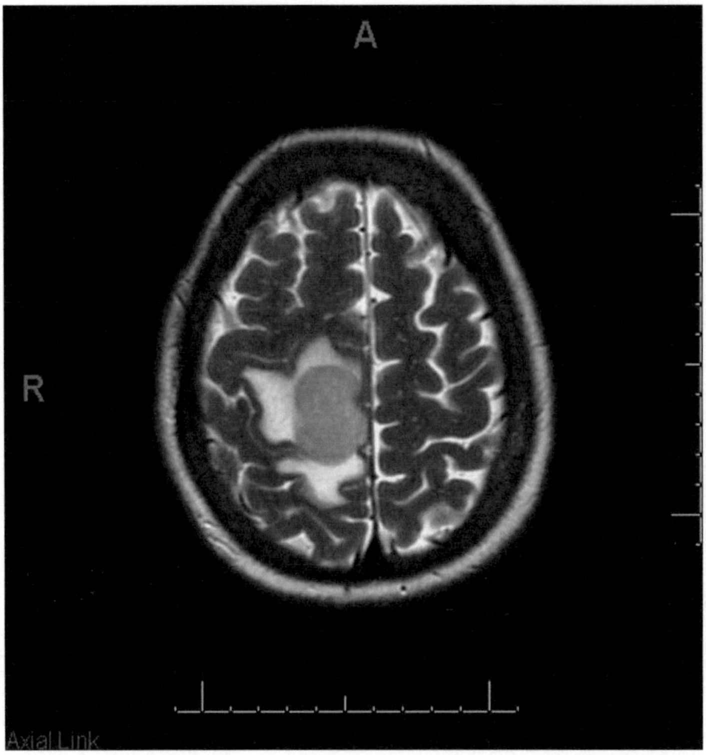

Figures 2–6. MRI of the brain, initial presentation. Axial T2, DWI/ADC, T1, T1 postcontrast, coronal T1 postcontrast. Right centrum semioval focal intra-axial mass is shown. The lesion is hypointense in T2, with vasogenic edema (Figure 2), restricted diffusion (Figure 3), and hypo-T1 (Figure 4) with homogeneous enhancement (Figures 5 and 6). MRI appearance is suggestive of hypercellularity (low T2, low ADC) as seen in CNS lymphoma.

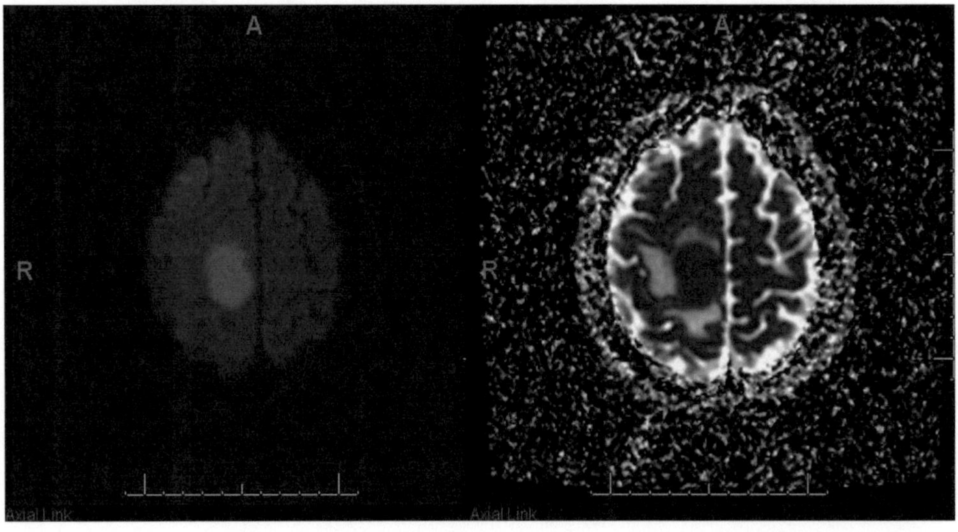

Figure 3.

http://dx.doi.org/10.5772/66601

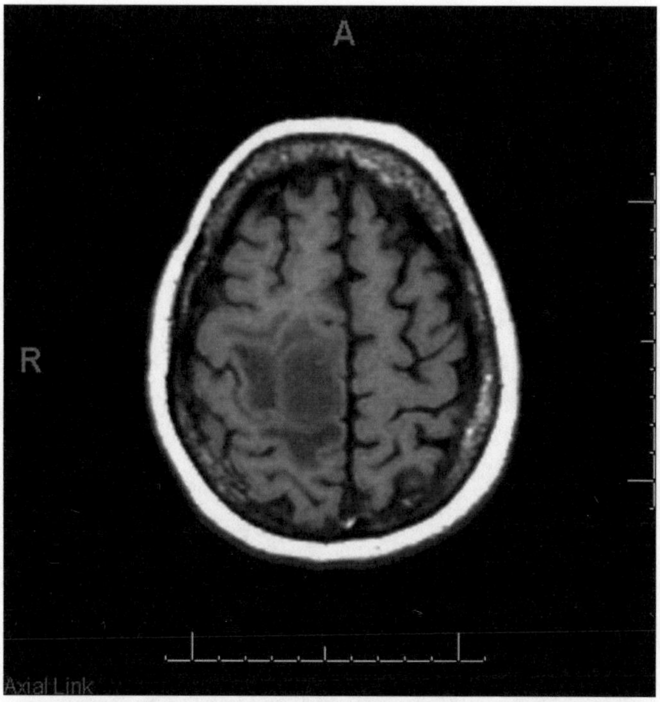

Figure 4.

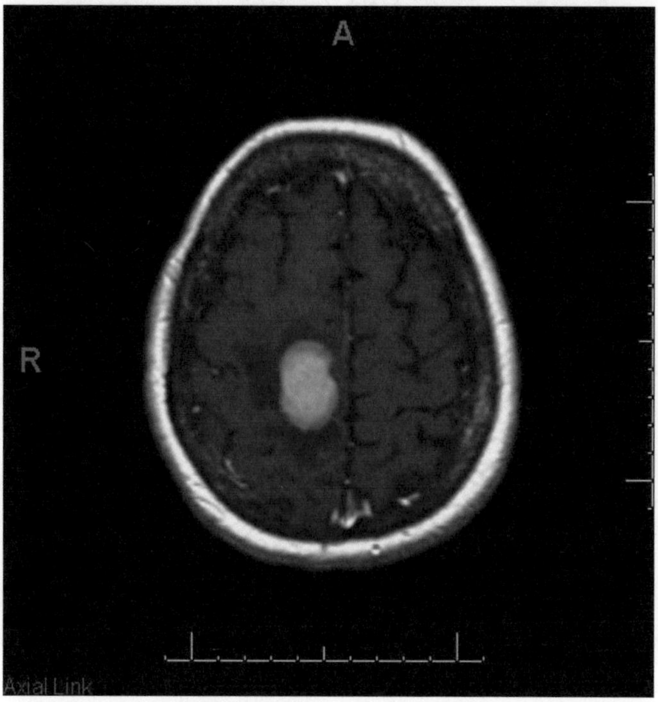

Figure 5.

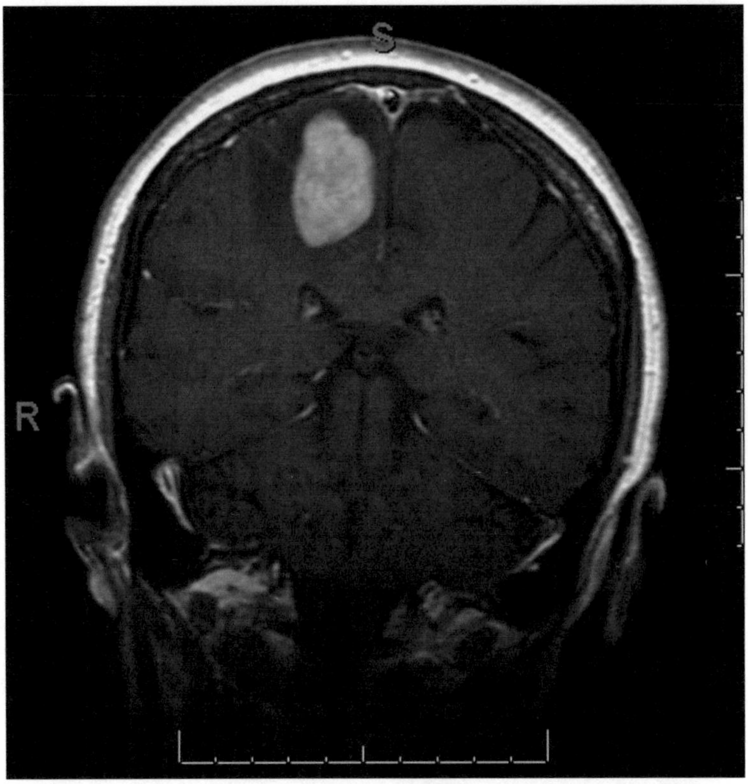

Figure 6.

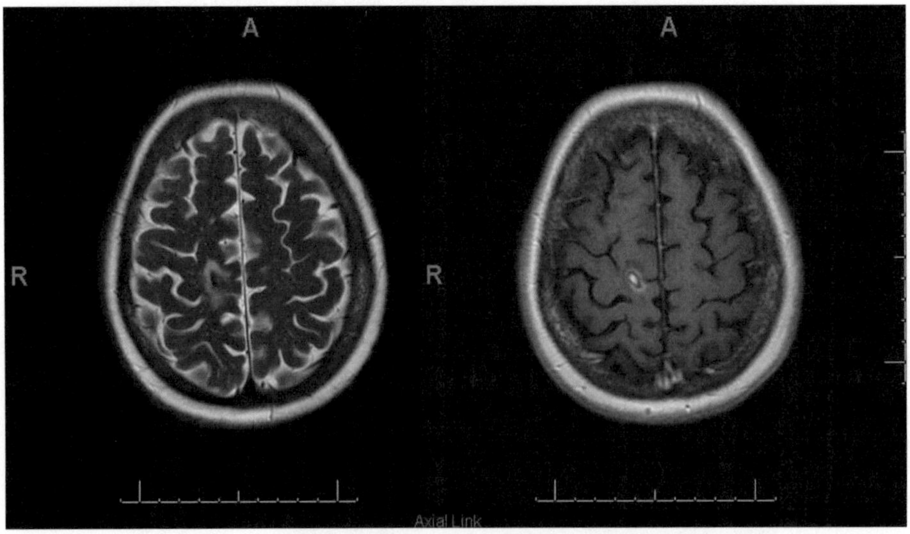

Figure 7. Follow up MRI of the brain at 3 months (post-HD-MTX and rituximab treatment). Axial T2, T1 postcontrast. Excellent treatment response with nearly complete resolution of the initial lesion. Please note the presence of small amounts of products within the lesion related to the initial stereotactic biopsy.

http://dx.doi.org/10.5772/66601

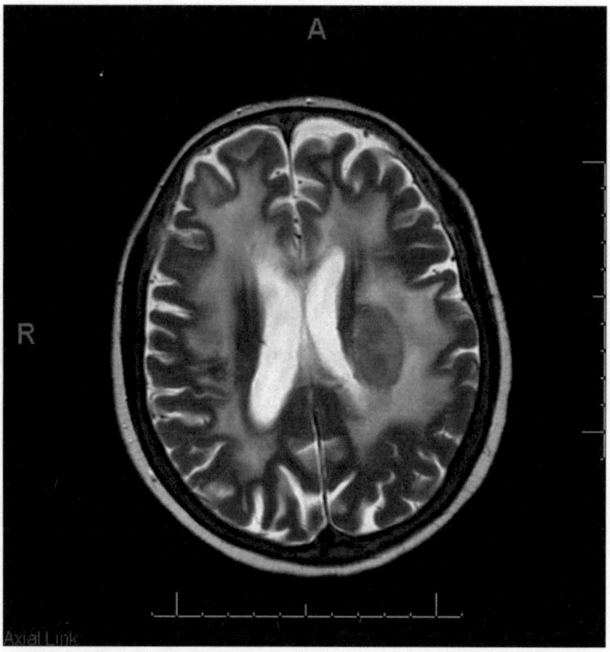

Figures 8–10. Brain MRI axial T2, T1 with contrast. Recurrence at 18 months, post-HD-MTX/rituximab/temozolomide and whole-brain radiation treatment. Bilateral tumor recurrence, with new lesions, similar in MRI appearance to the initial lesion. Please note the typical distribution in the deep hemispheric white matter and near the corpus callosum. Please note extensive diffuse postradiation white matter changes.

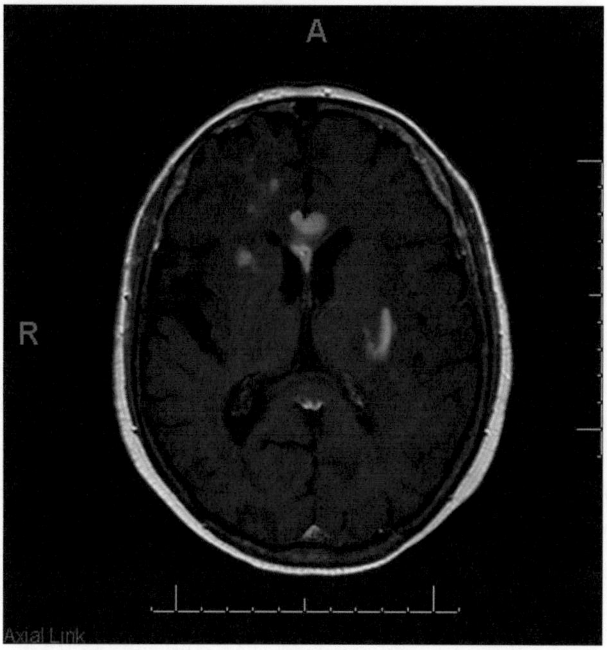

Figure 9.

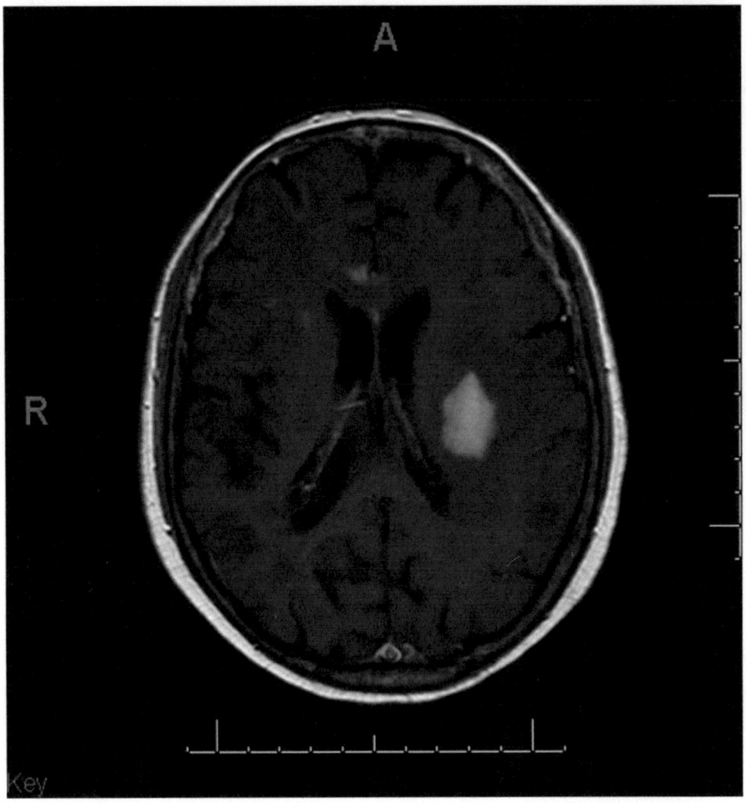

Figure 10.

Eye slit lamp examination is an integral part of the tumor extension workup, because of the frequent ocular involvement, and can prompt for subsequent imaging approaches like MRI. Also, if eye examination is positive for involvement, a vitreous biopsy can replace the brain biopsy and allow for a positive diagnosis.

Corticospinal fluid (CSF) examination by lumbar puncture should be performed in cases where it can be performed safely, which represents the majority of patients, as judged by the imaging and eye examinations. Cytology of CSF is rarely positive in PCNSL. However, cytologic and flow cytometric examination, as well as clonality assays, is warranted, and if evidence for lymphoma is strong enough by this approach, the brain lesion biopsy may become unnecessary. Also, there are new proposals for diagnostic approaches, which investigate CSF levels of interleukin (IL)-10, CXCL13, or micro RNAs (miRs) to sustain the suspicion of lymphoma, currently under investigation [23].

Histological examination of a tumor biopsy is the standard diagnostic approach. Biopsies should be as noninvasive as possible, and stereotactic biopsy is the best choice. Large tumor excision does not improve disease prognosis, can lead to significant neurologic sequelae, and also can delay the onset of treatment because of the surgical trauma and the risk of complications.

Laboratory tests include:

—Full blood count plus differential.

—Viral testing: HIV (mandatory, because of an increased PCNSL incidence in HIV-infected patients), hepatitis B and hepatitis C (especially if administration of immunotherapy is contemplated which can lead to viral reactivation or flaring).

—Basic pretherapeutic blood biochemistry to evaluate chemotherapy tolerance: liver function tests, kidney function, and electrolytes. Lactate dehydrogenase levels are of prognostic significance.

3.1. Staging and prognostic markers

There currently is no dedicated staging system for PCNSL. Using the Ann Arbor staging, PCNSL is usually a stage IEA lymphoma and as such is of limited clinical relevance. Prognostic indices commonly employed are the International Prognostic Index (IPI) and age-adjusted IPI, both including staging as a criterium. The International Extranodal Lymphoma Study Group has proposed a prognostic score for PCNSL based on five parameters: age>60 years, ECOG performance status>1, increased lactate dehydrogenases, elevated CSF protein levels, and deep brain localization of the tumor and proposed three prognostic groups: good risk (0–1 factors present), intermediate risk (2–3 factors), and high risk (3–4 factors). Although at the time of publication, in 2003, this score could discriminate well the outcomes of the three groups, it is of limited clinical use, because of the scarcity of therapeutic options limiting treatment adaptation according to the calculated score.

Performance status either according to ECOG/WHO or Karnofsky performance status scale is a useful indicator of the patient's tolerance profile for aggressive approaches and may help in the adaptation of dose intensity of therapeutic regimens.

4. Treatment of PCNSL

Prognosis of PCNSL is dismal, and therapeutic results are rather poor, especially when compared to other aggressive lymphomas. The outcome has witnessed a constant improvement over the last decades. As with other malignancies, it is unclear to what extent this improvement can be credited to a progress in anticancer agents, which have not dramatically changed for PCNSL until recently and how much of the progress should rather be attributed to a constant improvement in supportive measures, including the management of treatment-related complications. The development of better antibiotics and antifungals, as well as the advent of hematopoietic stimulating agents, allowed for drug dose and regimen intensity escalations and reduced treatment-related mortality, which could explain the ascending trend of therapeutic results.

As with other hematologic cancers, the treatment paradigm of PCNSL involves the induction of a complete remission (CR), followed by consolidation strategies aimed at preventing disease recurrence. Radiotherapy was, historically, the first nonsurgical therapeutic approach in lymphoma. Due to the particularities of CNS lymphoma, whole-brain radiotherapy (WBRT) is the standard radiation therapy approach and may include a boost to the involved CNS area. Unfortunately, WBRT is not only highly ineffective in curing lymphoma outside a combination with systemic treatment, but it is also associated with severe immediate and delayed neurotoxicity, including alteration of cognitive functions, sometimes severe and irreversible.

The addition of methotrexate (MTX)-based Systemic therapy has allowed in the 1970s for a significant improvement in cerebral lymphoma outcome, while the classical combination chemotherapy is used for nodal NHL, consisting of CHOP or CHOP-like regimens, demonstrating unsatisfactory results in PCNSL [26]. The standard first-line regimens today are constantly including high-dose MTX (HD-MTX) as the backbone of chemotherapy. MTX, aracytine; alkylating agents like busulfan, carmustine, lomustine, thiotepa, and ifosfamide; and platinum compounds have demonstrated their ability to cross the blood-brain barrier in efficient amounts. Although the CNS/CSF to plasma ratio for systemic MTX is low at around 5%, the CNS penetrance is sufficient for achieving therapeutic results but only at high systemic doses which usually start at 1.5 g/m^2 and go up to above 8g/m^2 [27]. An algorithm of the typical frontline treatment of PCNSL is presented in **Figure 11**.

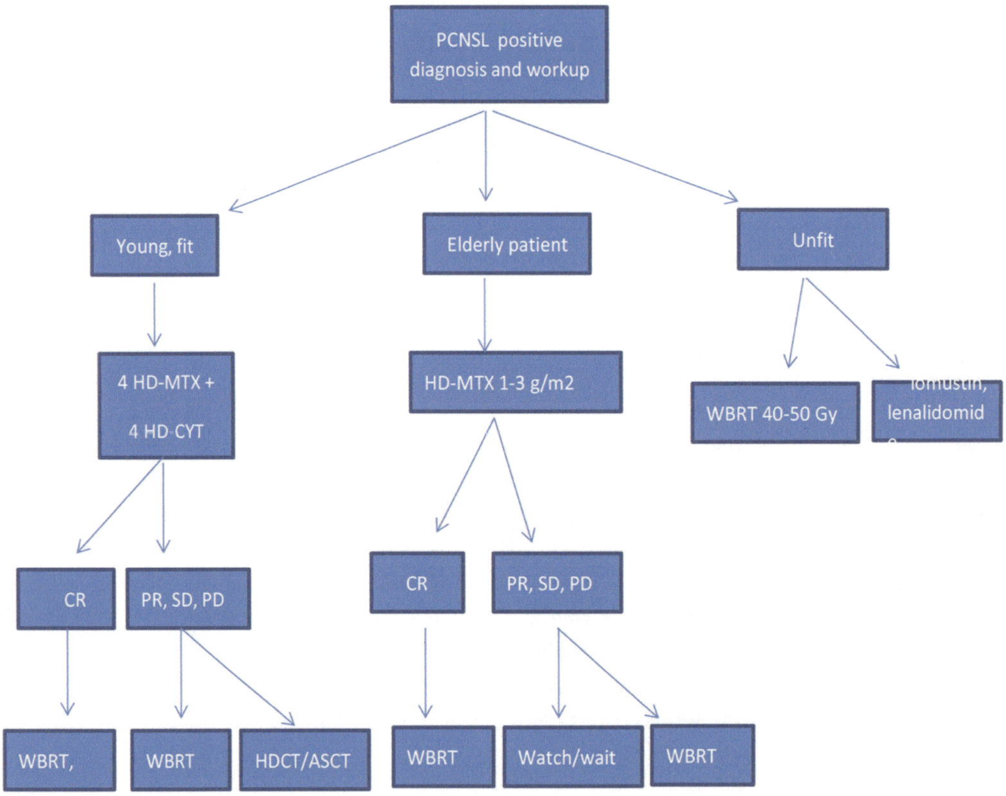

Figure 11. Treatment algorithm for newly diagnosed patients, according to the National Comprehensive Cancer Network [45] and European Society for Medical Oncology [29] evidence-based guidelines.

4.1. First-line induction therapy

The remission induction treatment for PCNSL is chemotherapy based, with anti-CD20 immunotherapy being added in recent years. MTX, which had been previously used in high doses with leucovorin rescue in the management of CNS involvement of acute lymphoblastic leukemia has been reported as efficient in CNS lymphoma, either primary or secondary to systemic disease, in the late 1970s, at doses ranging from 1 to 7.5 g/m^2. Subsequently, HD-MTX became the backbone of PCNSL induction therapy and currently used doses which range from 3 to 8 g/m^2, and it was demonstrated that systemic MTX at doses over 3.5 g/m^2 alleviates the need for concomitant intrathecal administration of the drug [6, 28]. Although a great step forward in PCNSL, single-agent MTX achieved complete remission (CR) rates of only approximately 30% as frontline induction therapy [29]. The addition of cytarabine to MTX allowed for an improvement of CR rates to 46% versus 18% with MTX as single agent with an overall response rate of 69% versus 40% in one of the few randomized prospective studies performed [26]. The addition of alkylating agents or vincristine to MTX and cytarabine did not alter induction treatment efficiency [29, 30]. The optimal number of cycles of induction chemotherapy is not clearly established, but six to eight two-weekly administrations are currently used [6]. For the frail or elderly patients not able to withstand intensive regimens, alkylating agents like temozolomide and lomustine are proposed, with temozolomide achieving CR rates of nearly 50%, comparable to HD-MTX-based regimens [31].

Association of immunotherapy with anti-CD20 antibodies, which greatly improves outcomes in nodal B-cell NHL, was not expected to be efficient in PCNSL, as rituximab is a macromolecule unable to bypass the blood-brain barrier (BBB). CSF concentrations of rituximab are normally less than 1% of systemic concentrations but can reach higher levels when coadministered with chemotherapy possibly due to BBB disruption. Inclusion of rituximab in the induction therapy of PCNSL has yielded controversial results and is not a current evidence-based guideline recommended standard practice, but is routinely used by many hematologists. Another approach currently under investigation is the intrathecal administration of rituximab, either by lumbar puncture or via an Ommaya reservoir. Adjunction of rituximab to chemotherapy was reported to significantly improve PCNSL outcome in a recently published retrospective study [32], and one of the largest prospective randomized studies in PCNSL, including 227 patients of up to 70 years of age, recently reported preliminary results showing that rituximab with or without thiotepa, plus HD-MTX and cytarabine, achieved superior remission rates as compared to HD-MTX and cytarabine alone, and the authors proposed the thiotepa, rituximab, plus HD-MTX and cytarabine (MATRix) regimen as the new standard induction regimen for fit patients [33]. Qian et al. reported interesting results with R-IDARAM in combination with intrathecal chemotherapy for newly diagnosed PCNSL patients. Treatment consisted of six cycles, administered at 3 weeks of interval, of rituximab 375 mg/m^2 (day 1), idarubicin 10 mg/m^2 (day 2 and 3), dexamethasone 100 mg/m^2 (12 h infusion on days 2, 3, and 4), cytarabine 1 g/m^2 (1 h. infusion on days 2 and 3), MTX 2 g/m^2 (6 h infusion on day 4 with folinic acid rescue), intrathecal rituximab 10 mg, MTX 15 mg, dexamethasone 5 mg ,and cytarabine 50 mg once a week. The reported CR rate for the 19 patients treated was an impressive 89% [34].

4.2. Consolidation therapy

Initially used as the single available therapeutic approach besides tumor excision, WBRT in dosed of 40–45 Gy became the standard consolidation regimen after the advent of methotrexate-based therapies. WBRT is a side effect-ridden approach, with high risk of neurotoxicity including cognition and memory impairment, brain atrophy, leukoencephalopathy, dementia, and endocrine abnormalities estimated at 25–35% at 5 years and up to 30% mortality rate [30, 35].

Dahlborg et al. published in 1996 what they called a first example of a durable response in PCNSL patients with chemotherapy alone, reporting, in a 58 PCNSL patient cohort retrospective analysis, similar results in patients treated with chemotherapy alone versus WBRT followed by chemotherapy [36]. Since, there has been a continuous quest for improving systemic therapy to alleviate the need for brain irradiation. Although the advent of combination chemotherapy rendered radiotherapy obsolete in many types of lymphoma, it is still an integral part of some currently employed treatment regimens, especially in Hodgkin's lymphomas and their histologically close relative, primary mediastinal B-cell lymphoma. In PCNSL, WBRT including the eyes is used because the diffuse infiltrative pattern of lymphoma, with focal radiotherapy resulting in a higher recurrence rate. Higher doses of irradiation did not improve the results and was associated with more severe neurotoxicity. A meta-analysis was published in 2001 investigating radiotherapy and optimal induction chemotherapy in PCNSL; radiation doses higher than 40 Gy did not show improved OS, and there was no outcome difference between immediate and delayed consolidation WBRT in patients achieving CR after chemotherapy [37]. As results of trials investigating the omission of radiotherapy as a consolidation therapeutic modality are conflicting, to date there are no definitive answers to this question. The majority of local protocols omit, however, WBRT as part of the first-line treatment of PCNSL, but its importance in relapsed/refractory disease is clearly established [5]. Also, WBRT at doses of 40–50 Gy is an option for patients where chemotherapy is contraindicated. In patients with the usual DLBCL aggressive histology, this strategy has a merely palliative role, with a chance of CR of less than 20% and short overall survival. However, in patients with the rarer, indolent lymphoma histology including marginal zone, lymphoplasmacytic, lymphocytic, plasmocytoma, and Hodgkin's, WBRT can be used with curative intent.

4.3. Bone marrow transplantation

High-dose chemotherapy followed by autologous stem cell transplantation (HDCT/ASCT) is usually reserved for the relapsed/refractory setting. The 2-year overall survival rate is less than 50%. Usually, conditioning regimens are thiotepa based and busulfan based, but the BEAM conditioning regimen typically employed for nodal lymphomas is still used in PCNSL, despite its low BBB penetrance. HDCT/ASCT has been recently investigated as a consolidation therapy after high-dose MTX-based regimens, particularly to avoid the neurological risk of WBRT. There are ongoing trials to establish the role of ASCT as first-line consolidation therapy [38].

4.4. Second-line/salvage therapy

If the long-term disease-free survival in newly diagnosed PCNSL approaches 50%, in relapsed/refractory disease, the CR and overall survival rates are discouraging, and there

http://dx.doi.org/10.5772/66601

currently is no standard of care. Ideally, the second-line therapy should employ agents not used in frontline treatment and be followed by ASCT. If the first remission was longer than 12 months, HD-MTX-based re-induction can be attempted, followed by either autologous transplantation or WBRT, depending on which of those has been used in the frontline approach

Alkylating agents such as temozolomide, thiotepa, or lomustine with or without rituximab are another therapeutic option in this setting. Like with all cancers, patient inclusion on a clinical trial is highly recommended. Novel therapeutic approaches, some of which are discussed below, are either under investigation or in development, in a disease group where therapy represents a major unmet of current hematologic clinical practice.

4.5. Novel approaches in PCNSL treatment

Ibrutinib is a novel agent acting as a covalent Bruton tyrosine kinase inhibitor, belonging to the B-cell receptor signaling inhibitors and showing remarkable activity in B-cell malignancy. It has been approved by the Food and Drug Administration and the European Medicines Agency in chronic lymphocytic leukemia, mantle cell lymphoma, and Waldenstrom's macroglobulinemia, and trials in other B-cell malignancies are ongoing. Ibrutinib was shown to penetrate the blood-brain barrier and to be active in cerebral involvement of mantle cell lymphoma and Waldenstrom's macroglobulinemia [39, 40]. Recently, preliminary results in relapsed/refractory PCNSL and secondary CNS lymphoma were available from a phase I study, where, in a small group of 10 patients, the drug demonstrated a good tolerance profile and an overall response rate of 78% [41].

Lenalidomide and other immunomodulatory drugs. After thalidomide, the infamous sedative drug withdrawn during the 1970s because of its teratogenic effects, was reinvented as an effective and well-tolerated anti-myeloma oral drug two decades ago, spice-up successors like lenalidomide and pomalidomide with better anti-myeloma activity and less side effects were developed. Although their efficacy was initially credited to anti-neoangiogenetic effects, hampering tumor growth, other immune-enhancing pathways of action were subsequently characterized, and the class is currently referred to as immunomodulatory drugs (IMiDs) and was shown to be active not only in B-cell malignancies but also in particular myeloproliferative neoplasms and myelodysplastic syndromes. Lenalidomide has shown efficacy in aggressive B-cell lymphomas like DLBCL or mantle cell lymphoma and also as a graft-versus-disease enhancer in the post-allogeneic transplantation setting. Lenalidomide has the advantage of a good safety profile and tolerance, making it extremely useful in elderly or frail patients, not able to withstand intensive therapeutic approaches [42]. Lenalidomide is being investigated in PCNSL and has been shown to penetrate the BBB, with good intraventricular, intraocular, and brain tissue penetrance. Lenalidomide has been administered either as a single agent or in combination with systemic or intraventricular rituximab. Although efficacy of lenalidomide was only reported in isolated case reports or small case series and phase I trials, it seems to be an interesting agent credited with great expectations especially in the frail PCNSL patients where therapeutic options are extremely limited [43, 44].

5. Conclusions

PCNSL is presently one of the deadliest lymphomas, with a cure rate estimated as being lower than 50%, and therapeutic improvement lags behind that of nodal lymphomas due to the rarity of the disease, making patient accrual for prospective studies difficult. There is ongoing controversy about the pathobiology of PCNSL, and consensus evidence-based guidelines for its management are difficult to formulate. The current treatment for PCNSL consists of combination chemotherapy with a high-dose methotrexate-based backbone. Brain radiotherapy has demonstrated its efficiency as a consolidation regimen, but newer approaches tend to avoid radiotherapy and replace it with chemoimmunotherapy including high-dose therapy with autologous stem cell support, because of the serious side effects of the former. Despite significant progress, PCNSL therapy remains a major unmet for hematologists, and the development of new therapeutic approaches is warranted.

Acknowledgements

This work was supported by a grant from the Romanian National Authority for Scientific Research and Innovation, CNCS—UEFISCDI, project number PN-II-RU-TE-2014-4-2074 to Drs. MZ and CB.

Author details

Mihnea Zdrenghea[1, 2*], Delia Dima[2], Ciprian Tomuleasa[1, 2], Horia Bumbea[3] and Cristina Bagacean[1, 4]

*Address all correspondence to: mzdrenghea@umfcluj.ro

1 Department of Hematology, Iuliu Hatieganu University of Medicine and Pharmacy, Cluj-Napoca, Romania

2 Department of Hematology, Ion Chiricuta Oncology Institute, Cluj-Napoca, Romania

3 Department of Hematology, Carol Davila University of Medicine and Pharmacy, Bucharest, Romania

4 Laboratory of Immunology and Immunotherapy, Brest University Medical School, CHRU Morvan, Brest, France

References

[1] Hoffman S, Propp JM, McCarthy BJ. Temporal trends in incidence of primary brain tumors in the United States, 1985–1999. Neuro Oncol. 2006 Jan;8(1):27-37.

[2] Rubenstein J, Ferreri AJ, Pittaluga S. Primary lymphoma of the central nervous system: epidemiology, pathology and current approaches to diagnosis, prognosis and treatment. Leuk Lymphoma. 2008;49(Suppl 1):43-51.

[3] Ferreri AJ, Marturano E. Primary CNS lymphoma. Best Pract Res Clin Haematol. 2012 Mar;25(1):119-130.

[4] Swerdlow SH, Campo E, Pileri SA, Harris NL, Stein H, Siebert R, et al. The 2016 revision of the World Health Organization classification of lymphoid neoplasms. Blood. 2016 May 19;127(20):2375-2390.

[5] DeAngelis LM. Whither whole brain radiotherapy for primary CNS lymphoma? Neuro Oncol. 2014 Aug;16(8):1032-1034.

[6] Fraser E, Gruenberg K, Rubenstein JL. New approaches in primary central nervous system lymphoma. Chin Clin Oncol. 2015 Mar;4(1):11.

[7] Ferreri AJ, Reni M, Pasini F, Calderoni A, Tirelli U, Pivnik A, et al. A multicenter study of treatment of primary CNS lymphoma. Neurology. 2002 May 28;58(10):1513-1520.

[8] Tu PH, Giannini C, Judkins AR, Schwalb JM, Burack R, O'Neill BP, et al. Clinicopathologic and genetic profile of intracranial marginal zone lymphoma: a primary low-grade CNS lymphoma that mimics meningioma. J Clin Oncol. 2005 Aug 20;23(24):5718-5727.

[9] Montesinos-Rongen M, Kuppers R, Schluter D, Spieker T, Van Roost D, Schaller C, et al. Primary central nervous system lymphomas are derived from germinal-center B cells and show a preferential usage of the V4-34 gene segment. Am J Pathol. 1999 Dec;155(6):2077-2086.

[10] Larocca LM, Capello D, Rinelli A, Nori S, Antinori A, Gloghini A, et al. The molecular and phenotypic profile of primary central nervous system lymphoma identifies distinct categories of the disease and is consistent with histogenetic derivation from germinal center-related B cells. Blood. 1998 Aug 1;92(3):1011-1019.

[11] Thompsett AR, Ellison DW, Stevenson FK, Zhu D. V(H) gene sequences from primary central nervous system lymphomas indicate derivation from highly mutated germinal center B cells with ongoing mutational activity. Blood. 1999 Sep 1;94(5):1738-1746.

[12] Camilleri-Broet S, Criniere E, Broet P, Delwail V, Mokhtari K, Moreau A, et al. A uniform activated B-cell-like immunophenotype might explain the poor prognosis of primary central nervous system lymphomas: analysis of 83 cases. Blood. 2006 Jan 1;107(1):190-196.

[13] Rubenstein JL, Hsi ED, Johnson JL, Jung SH, Nakashima MO, Grant B, et al. Intensive chemotherapy and immunotherapy in patients with newly diagnosed primary CNS lymphoma: CALGB 50202 (Alliance 50202). J Clin Oncol. 2013 Sep 1;31(25):3061-3068.

[14] Fischer L, Hummel M, Korfel A, Lenze D, Joehrens K, Thiel E. Differential micro-RNA expression in primary CNS and nodal diffuse large B-cell lymphomas. Neuro Oncol. 2011 Oct;13(10):1090-1098.

[15] Cady FM, O'Neill BP, Law ME, Decker PA, Kurtz DM, Giannini C, et al. Del(6)(q22) and BCL6 rearrangements in primary CNS lymphoma are indicators of an aggressive clinical course. J Clin Oncol. 2008 Oct 10;26(29):4814-4819.

[16] Harada K, Nishizaki T, Kubota H, Suzuki M, Sasaki K. Distinct primary central nervous system lymphoma defined by comparative genomic hybridization and laser scanning cytometry. Cancer Genet Cytogenet. 2001 Mar;125(2):147-150.

[17] Boonstra R, Koning A, Mastik M, van den Berg A, Poppema S. Analysis of chromosomal copy number changes and oncoprotein expression in primary central nervous system lymphomas: frequent loss of chromosome arm 6q. Virchows Arch. 2003 Aug;443(2):164-169.

[18] Montesinos-Rongen M, Schmitz R, Brunn A, Gesk S, Richter J, Hong K, et al. Mutations of CARD11 but not TNFAIP3 may activate the NF-kappaB pathway in primary CNS lymphoma. Acta Neuropathol. 2010 Oct;120(4):529-535.

[19] Gonzalez-Aguilar A, Idbaih A, Boisselier B, Habbita N, Rossetto M, Laurenge A, et al. Recurrent mutations of MYD88 and TBL1XR1 in primary central nervous system lymphomas. Clin Cancer Res. 2012 Oct 1;18(19):5203-5211.

[20] Campo E, Swerdlow SH, Harris NL, Pileri S, Stein H, Jaffe ES. The 2008 WHO classification of lymphoid neoplasms and beyond: evolving concepts and practical applications. Blood. 2011 May 12;117(19):5019-5032.

[21] Louis DN, Ohgaki H, Wiestler OD, Cavenee WK, Burger PC, Jouvet A, et al. The 2007 WHO classification of tumours of the central nervous system. Acta Neuropathol. 2007 Aug;114(2):97-109.

[22] Smith JR, Braziel RM, Paoletti S, Lipp M, Uguccioni M, Rosenbaum JT. Expression of B-cell-attracting chemokine 1 (CXCL13) by malignant lymphocytes and vascular endothelium in primary central nervous system lymphoma. Blood. 2003 Feb 1;101(3):815-821.

[23] Rubenstein JL, Wong VS, Kadoch C, Gao HX, Barajas R, Chen L, et al. CXCL13 plus interleukin 10 is highly specific for the diagnosis of CNS lymphoma. Blood. 2013 Jun 6;121(23):4740-4748.

[24] Louveau A, Smirnov I, Keyes TJ, Eccles JD, Rouhani SJ, Peske JD, et al. Structural and functional features of central nervous system lymphatic vessels. Nature. 2015 Jul 16;523(7560):337-341.

[25] Sagoo MS, Mehta H, Swampillai AJ, Cohen VM, Amin SZ, Plowman PN, et al. Primary intraocular lymphoma. Surv Ophthalmol. 2014 Sep-Oct;59(5):503-516.

[26] Ferreri AJ, Reni M, Foppoli M, Martelli M, Pangalis GA, Frezzato M, et al. High-dose cytarabine plus high-dose methotrexate versus high-dose methotrexate alone in patients with primary CNS lymphoma: a randomised phase 2 trial. Lancet. 2009 Oct 31;374(9700):1512-1520.

[27] Korfel A. A focus on pharmacotherapy for primary central nervous system lymphoma. Expert Rev Hematol. 2015 Oct;8(5):559-562.

[28] Khan RB, Shi W, Thaler HT, DeAngelis LM, Abrey LE. Is intrathecal methotrexate necessary in the treatment of primary CNS lymphoma? J Neurooncol. 2002 Jun;58(2):175-178.

[29] Vitolo U, Seymour JF, Martelli M, Illerhaus G, Illidge T, Zucca E, et al. Extranodal diffuse large B-cell lymphoma (DLBCL) and primary mediastinal B-cell lymphoma: ESMO Clinical Practice Guidelines for diagnosis, treatment and follow-up. Ann Oncol. 2016 Sep;27(suppl 5):v91-v102.

[30] Shah GD, Yahalom J, Correa DD, Lai RK, Raizer JJ, Schiff D, et al. Combined immunochemotherapy with reduced whole-brain radiotherapy for newly diagnosed primary CNS lymphoma. J Clin Oncol. 2007 Oct 20;25(30):4730-4735.

[31] Kurzwelly D, Glas M, Roth P, Weimann E, Lohner H, Waha A, et al. Primary CNS lymphoma in the elderly: temozolomide therapy and MGMT status. J Neurooncol. 2010 May;97(3):389-392.

[32] Mocikova H, Pytlik R, Sykorova A, Janikova A, Prochazka V, Vokurka S, et al. Role of rituximab in treatment of patients with primary central nervous system lymphoma: a retrospective analysis of the Czech lymphoma study group registry. Leuk Lymphoma. 2016 Dec;57(12):2777-2783.

[33] Ferreri AJ, Cwynarski K, Pulczynski E, Ponzoni M, Deckert M, Politi LS, et al. Chemoimmunotherapy with methotrexate, cytarabine, thiotepa, and rituximab (MATRix regimen) in patients with primary CNS lymphoma: results of the first randomisation of the International Extranodal Lymphoma Study Group-32 (IELSG32) phase 2 trial. Lancet Haematol. 2016 May;3(5):e217-e227.

[34] Qian L, Zhou C, Shen J, Cen J, Yin W. Treatment of newly diagnosed B-cell origin primary CNS lymphoma with systemic R-IDARAM chemotherapy and intrathecal immunochemotherapy. Oncotarget. 2016 May 3;7(18):25783-25790.

[35] Abrey LE, DeAngelis LM, Yahalom J. Long-term survival in primary CNS lymphoma. J Clin Oncol. 1998 Mar;16(3):859-863.

[36] Dahlborg SA, Henner WD, Crossen JR, Tableman CM, Petrillo A, Braziel R, et al. Non-AIDS primary CNS lymphoma: first example of a durable response in a primary brain tumor using enhanced chemotherapy delivery without cognitive loss and without radiotherapy. Cancer J Sci Am. 1996 May-Jun;2(3):166-174.

[37] Reni M, Ferreri AJ, Guha-Thakurta N, Blay JY, Dell'Oro S, Biron P, et al. Clinical relevance of consolidation radiotherapy and other main therapeutic issues in primary central nervous system lymphomas treated with upfront high-dose methotrexate. Int J Radiat Oncol Biol Phys. 2001 Oct 1;51(2):419-425.

[38] Ferreri AJ, Illerhaus G. The role of autologous stem cell transplantation in primary central nervous system lymphoma. Blood. 2016 Mar 31;127(13):1642-1649.

[39] Mason C, Savona S, Rini JN, Castillo JJ, Xu L, Hunter ZR, et al. Ibrutinib penetrates the blood brain barrier and shows efficacy in the therapy of Bing Neel syndrome. Br J Haematol. doi:10.1111/bjh.14218.

[40] Bernard S, Goldwirt L, Amorim S, Brice P, Briere J, de Kerviler E, et al. Activity of ibrutinib in mantle cell lymphoma patients with central nervous system relapse. Blood. 2015 Oct 1;126(14):1695-1698.

[41] Grommes C, Kaley T, Craig N, Padula Omuro A, Wolfe J, Mellinghoff I, et al. Phase I study of single agent ibrutinib in recurrent/refractory primary (PCNSL) and secondary CNS lymphoma (SCNSL). J Clinical Oncol. [Abstract]. 2016;34(15):Abstract 2046.

[42] Tempescul A, Ianotto JC, Bagacean C, Salaun PY, Bocsan C, Zdrenghea M. Late relapsing mantle cell lymphoma showing preserved sensitivity to single-agent lenalidomide. Int J Hematol. 2016 Sep;104(3):400-402.

[43] Rubenstein J, Formaker X, Wang X, Chen N, Seider M, Munster P, et al. Interim results of a phase I study of lenalidomide (CC-5013) plus intraventricular/intravenous rituximab for recurrent/refractory CNS and intraocular lymphoma. Blood. [Meeting abstract]. 2014; 124(56th ASH meeting abstracts):Abstract 4470.

[44] Houillier C, Choquet S, Touitou V, Martin-Duverneuil N, Navarro S, Mokhtari K, et al. Lenalidomide monotherapy as salvage treatment for recurrent primary CNS lymphoma. Neurology. 2015 Jan 20;84(3):325-326.

[45] NCCN Clinical Practice Guidelines in Oncology. Central Nervous System Cancers. 2016; Available from: www.nccn.org.

Section 7

New Drugs for CNS Malignancies

Chapter 9

Comparative Anticancer Activity in Human Tumor Xenograft Models, Preclinical Pharmacology and Toxicology for 4-Hydroperoxyifosfamide (HOOI): A Potential Neuro-Alkylating Agent for Primary and Metastatic Cancers Involving the Central Nervous System

Lee Roy Morgan, Andrew H. Rodgers,
Gerard Bastian, William S. Waud, Branko S. Jursic,
Robert F. Struck, Gerald LaHoste and
Edward Stevens

Additional information is available at the end of the chapter

http://dx.doi.org/10.5772/66304

Abstract

Background: 4-Hydropeoxyifosfamide (HOOI) is a hydroperoxy derivative of ifosfamide that was developed as an anticancer agent that can penetrate the blood-brain barrier (BBB), which can be potentially useful in the management of brain tumors.

Methods: A novel synthetic scheme for HOOI is presented and verified. HOOI and an HOOI L-lysine salt were prepared and mice implanted intracranially (IC) and in the mammary fat pad with human U251 glioblastoma, D54 glioblastoma, and MX-1 breast tumor xenografts and treated with HOOI IP once daily for 1–5 days. The animals were monitored for responses, increased long-term survival (ILS) and long-term survival (LTS). Mice, rats, and dogs received single IV doses of HOOI in a wide range of concentrations and results are compared and presented herein.

Results: HOOI has been synthesized as per a new route in 67% yield. The drug is stable when frozen in the absence of moisture; however, as a lysine salt the drug is stable in solution and as a lyophilized product. HOOI produced complete responses with improved long-term survival against IC implanted U251 glioblastoma, D54 glioblastoma, and MX-1 breast tumor xenografts in mice. The drug was superior to 4-demethyl-4-cholesteryloxycarbonylpenclomedine (DM-CHC-PEN) and BCNU vs. IC implanted tumor models. The HOOI lysine salt demonstrated equal activity to that of HOOI alone. Over all, the drug was well tolerated. Predictions for human pharmacokinetic parameters and dosing are made from allometric analysis using the above three species. Data predicted an acceptable starting dose of 39 mg/m^2 with a clearance of 11 L/h +/− 2.75 and a $T_{1/2\alpha}$ 15 min and $T_{½\beta}$ 5.30 h for a 70 kg human patient. The presented toxicity data plus strong antineuro-oncology activity supports DM-CHOC-PEN's proposed use as a treatment for CNS malignancies. The drug is being prepared for Phase I trial studies in the US–IND pending.

Keywords: HOOI, 4-hydroperoxyifosfamide, brain tumors, non-tumor target therapy, no renal toxicity

1. Introduction

Isophosphoramide mustard (IPM) (**Figure 1**) is the active metabolite of ifosfamide (IFOS) and a bifunctional DNA alkylator that generates guanine-cytosine interstrand cross-linking in G-X-C sequences producing cell death [1, 2]. Although IPM is the ultimate alkylator that is derived from IFOS, it has been removed from clinical trials because of lack of sufficient anticancer activity in clinical trials [3–5]. IFOS is still the phosphoramide mustard that is most used in sarcoma therapy; however, its use is hampered by requirement for hepatic activation and release of extracellular acrolein (ACR) and chloroacetaldehyde (CAA)—resulting in dose limiting cystitis, renal toxicity, and neurotoxicity, plus myelosuppression [6, 7].

4-Hydroperoxyifosfamide (HOOI, **Figure 1**) is a peroxide derivative of IFOS that spontaneously undergoes ring cleavage releasing acrolein and chloroacetaldehyde primarily *in situ* in cancer cells, not extracellularly in the general circulation as does IFOS [8–10]. The support data for HOOI's anticancer activity and toxicity is reviewed here.

DEKK-TEC's interest in HOOI was to document its potential usefulness as an anticancer agent and if it possesses any of IFOS' toxicities – cystitis, renal tubular necrosis, and CNS alterations, all of which hamper the usefulness and utilization of IFOS [6, 7]. A secondary goal was to develop a stable form of HOOI for clinical use [11, 12].

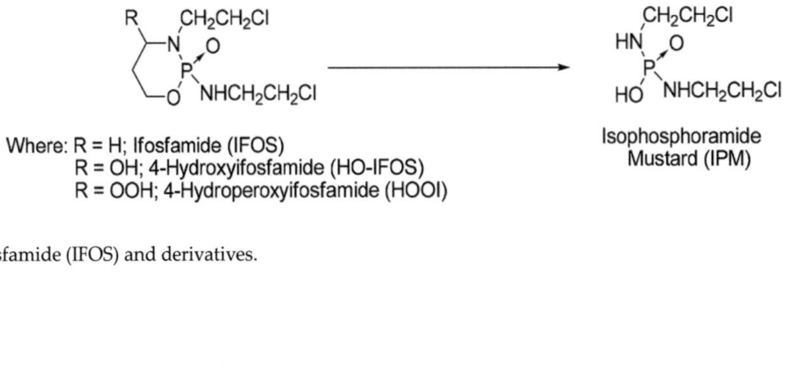

Figure 1. Ifosfamide (IFOS) and derivatives.

2. Chemistry, formulations and analyses

HOOI and the L-lysine salt have been synthesized at DEKK-TEC, Inc., using GLP/GMP guidelines, previously described in detail [8, 9, 13–16]. The HOOI-L-lysine salt is a very stable chemical in the solid state under ambient conditions, soluble in water or saline and can be administered to animals in a saline solution (10%); the elemental analysis, NMR, mass spectra, and X-ray crystallography all agreed with the structure given in **Figure 2** [9].

Bulk HOOI and the L-lysine salt are stable as a lyophilized powder and can be stored at 20–23°C for up to 1.6 years without deterioration [16].

HOOI is a weak acid which in prolonged contact with water undergoes hydrolysis resulting in IPM and deterioration; thus, the stability of HOOI has always been an issue [16]. The HOOI structure can be stabilized with L-lysine, a basic amino acid. The optimized structure for HOOI as the L-lysine salt is a ternary (three-molecule) HOOI-2-Lys complex—as described from molecular mechanics and semiempirical computational analysis of the HOOI-Lys complexes (**Figure 2**) [16]. Two lysine molecules aligned themselves "above" and "below" HOOI. L-lysine stabilizes the HOOI through hydrogen bonding between the –NH-PO-NH- moiety and the ammonium group of the lysine. In this way, the ternary complex prevents water molecules from approaching the acidic –NH–P=O moiety, thus protecting HOOI from hydrolysis [9, 11, 12, 16].

HOOI and its L-lysine salt (bulk, as well as, in aqueous solutions – including biological) can be assayed/monitored with standard high-pressure liquid chromatography (HPLC) analysis (**Figure 3**) [16].

However, the most useful method to monitor HOOI in biological samples (blood, urine, etc.) is with GC/MS [8, 16, 17]. HOOI can be derivatized with *t*-butyl dimethylsilyl-N-methyl-tri-

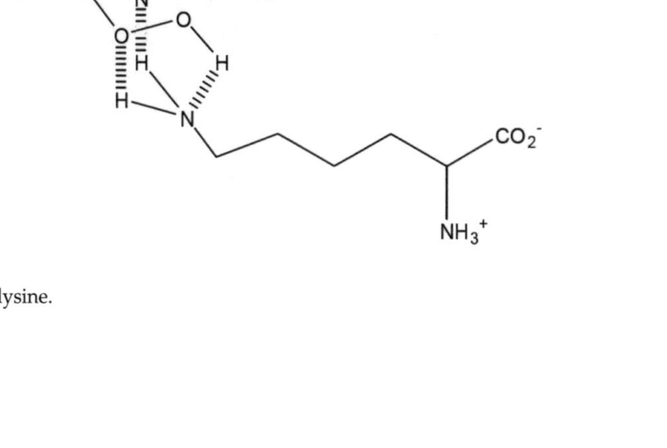

Figure 2. 4-HOOI/L-lysine.

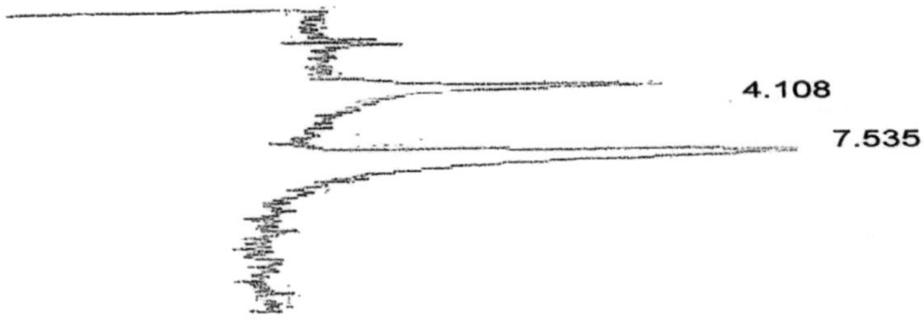

Figure 3. HPLC: retentions – L- lysine-4.018 and HOOI-7.535.

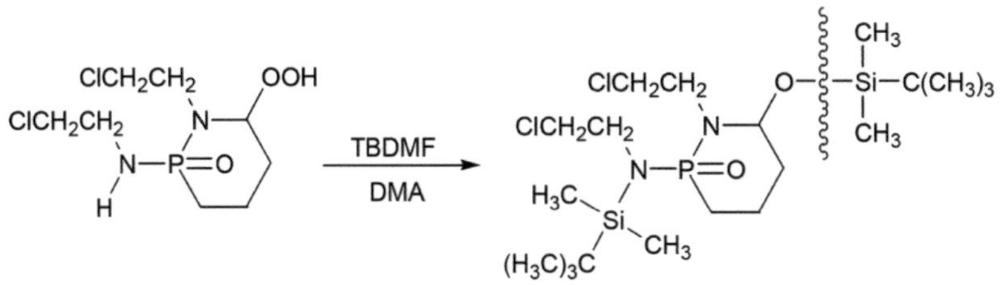

Figure 4. Derivatization of HOOI.

fluoroacetamide (TBDMF), which is very stable, easy to prepare, and reproducible in GC/MS assays (**Figure 4**) [8, 16, 17].

The GC/MS chromatogram for pure HOOI-TBDMF had a unique peak at 15 minutes. HOOI's quantification can be performed by selected ion monitoring (SIM) at $m/z = 406$ amu ($m = 520–114$) of fragments corresponding to the mass spectrum of the *t*-butyl dimethylsilyl derivatized compound revealing the loss of the well-known *t*-butyl dimethyl *Si* group (m-114) (**Figure 4**). Differences between HOOI and 4-HO-IFOS (a metabolite of IFOS, **Figure 1**) cannot be made on GC/MS, but this is resolved with HPLC [8, 9, 16].

The TBDMF derivatization of HOOI yield is 90% and limits of quantitation are 10 ng/mL; the extraction coefficients from plasma and saline are 75% and 98%, respectively [16]. Validation of the assay was conducted using GLP guidelines, with reference to the reported values per Struck et al. [12].

The GC/MS assay also allows identification of IPM (**Figure 1**), the ultimate degradation product and active anticancer species generated from both IFOS and HOOI [16].

3. Antitumor evaluation *in vivo*

Antitumor evaluations for HOOI were performed employing standard GLP guidelines at Southern Research Institute and DEKK-TEC [8, 9, 16, 18]. Human xenograft tumors (U251 or D54 human glioma) were implanted intracranially (IC) into athymic *NCr-nu/nu* and the 9L rat glioma implanted subcutaneously (SC) into *Hsd:SD* rats, respectively in concentrations of 10^6 cells per animal [16, 18]. All approved and monitored under the respective IACUCs.

Drug	Dose (mg/kg)	Life span (% ILS)	Long-term survival (% LTS)
Control	Vehicle	0	0/9
HOOI	100	+54	89% (8/9 CR)
HOOI·lys	125	+54	100% (9/9 CR)
IFOS	400	5	0
TMZ	120	+54	60% (3/5 CR)

Treatment Schedule: 8 days post-SC implant admin.
HOOI, IFOS—IP once; TMZ—PO q 4 day × 3. Species: Hsd:SD rats—female, Harlan rats; study termination at 54 days.

Table 1. Activities of HOOI and HOOI-Lys vs. 9L rat glioma in rat implant: 10^6 cells SC.

HOOI and the L-lysine salt were prepared as 10% saline solutions and evaluated against the above rodent tumor models per IP administered in doses ranges of 25–300 mg/kg per dose/day × 5 days, which included the maximum tolerated dose.

Of significance is that HOOI was curative at 90 mg/kg/day × 5 days (84% long-term survival, LTS, with 20% CR) against the human U251 glioblastoma implanted IC. In contrast BCNU—the gold standard for years in the treatment of gliomas produced—no CRs, while temozolamide (TMZ) [120 mg/kg/d × 3 days], the current standard produced identical responses to HOOI [16, 18, 19].

HOOI vs. HOOI-L-lysine salt possessed similar activity in a rat glioma model. No weight loss or hematuria was noted with either HOOI or the L-lysine salt. In contrast, IFOS produced gross hematuria; both HOOI and the L-lysine salt were well tolerated (**Table 1**).

4. Pharmacology and toxicity

The results for the acute IV toxicity studies for HOOI in mice and dogs are presented in **Tables 2** and **3**, which includes the median lethal dose values observed. Two separate single IV mouse-dosing studies calculated an $LD_{10/50}$ of 200/385 mg/kg (for both sexes; with 95% confidence limits) [16].

Route	Dose (mg/kg)	Number and sex	Observations
IV	0	5 M 5 F	No death
	50	5 M 5 F	No death
	100	5 M 5 F	No death
	200	5 M 5 F	0 M and 3 F—died
	300	5 M 5 F	4 M and 4 F—died
	400	5 M 5 F	5 M and 5 F—died

Table 2. Acute IV toxicity for HOOI in the mouse – DEKK-TEC study (Single dose).

Route/schedule	Dose (mg/kg)	Number and sex	Observations
IV once	0	2 M	No death
	10	2 M	No death
	15	2 M	No death
	20	2 M	All died
	30	2 M	All died

Table 3. Acute IV toxicity for HOOI in the dog.

Clinical deterioration occurred in both sexes of mice and rats post-HOOI dosing in a dose-dependent manner. No seizures or loss of coordination were observed [16].

4.1. Acute studies in mice

Table 2 reviews the acute toxicity for HOOI when administered intravenously in single doses of 50, 100, 150, 250, and 400 mg/kg to adult male and female mice, 10 animals per sex per dose level [16, 17, 19].

No animals died at 0, 100, or 150 mg/kg, then a dose vs. lethal response occurred (**Table 2**). The cause of death was generally from cardiovascular collapse. No seizures or CNS toxicities were reported. No macroscopic findings were reported in any of the animals [6, 19].

Based on the conditions and findings of this study, the intravenous LD_{10} of HOOI was calculated to be 200 mg/kg (95% confidence limits could not be calculated) in mice (combined sexes). Acute intravenous toxicity study results are presented in **Table 2**.

4.2. Acute intravenous toxicity in dogs [16]

A dog study evaluated the acute toxicity of HOOI, when administered via a single intravenous (bolus) injection to dogs (**Table 3**). Male beagle dogs, in groups of two (2) were administered HOOI at dose levels–10, 15, 20, and 30 mg/kg. One additional group of two male animals served as the control and received the vehicle, 0.9% sodium chloride, administered once on Day 1 via intravenous single bolus injection, at a dose volume of 1 mL/kg. Following administration, all animals were maintained on study for up to a 14-day observation period. Blood work was obtained for complete chemistry, hematological, and urine analyses, plus timed-blood samples for pharmacokinetic studies throughout the study.

No treatment-related effects were noted on coagulation, clinical chemistry, and urinalysis evaluations, or on macroscopic and organ weight evaluations during the study. Treatment related mortality was noted during the study, but was limited to the 20 and 30 mg/kg dose groups. All animals in these groups were euthanized *in extremis* on Day 8 due to their deteriorating physical condition and following veterinary consultation. The respective groups that were administered the vehicle control, HOOI—10 and 15 mg/kg, survived to their scheduled necropsy (Day 15).

Treatment-related clinical findings noted during the study were most prominent at 30 mg/kg and included decreased activity, feces few/absent, yellow discharge from the eyes, emesis/vomit, with decreased activity, and salivation which were also noted at 20 mg/kg. However, the animals in both these dose groups generally stopped (or nearly stopped) eating over time and would not respond to attempts to stimulate their appetite with canned food supplementary diet, leading to their continued deterioration and the need for subsequent early euthanasia *in extremis* on Day 8. At 15 mg/kg, some similar signs were seen (decreased activity, in appetence, and thinness in one animal; feces few/ absent in the other). The conditions of the latter dosed animals did not deteriorate over time (they responded to attempts to stimulate appetite with canned food supplementary diet), allowing them to survive to the scheduled necropsy on Day 15, as did the animals at 10 mg/kg, whose only noteworthy clinical finding was feces few/absent in one of the two animals [16]. Treatment-related body weight loss and correlated decreases in food consumption were noted at all HOOI dose levels, and exhibited a dose-response pattern of effect [16].

Alterations in hematology were noted as follows: erythrocytes, hemoglobin, and hematocrit decreased similarly in all treatment groups by Day 3, while the control animals tended to increase slightly. The erythrocytes and hematocrit tended to continue to decrease through Day 15 with the 15 mg/kg dose. At 10 mg/kg, there was little change in erythrocyte numbers of hemoglobin, but hematocrit continued to decrease slightly through Day 15. These changes in red cell parameters were accompanied by marked reductions of reticulocytes in treated animals, again with no dose-dependency. These reticulocytes were beginning to rebound at Day 15 in the surviving animals at 10 and 15 mg/kg. Total leukocytes tended to decrease slightly at 15 mg/kg by Day 3, and slightly more at 20 and 30 mg/kg. This was due primarily to dose-dependent decreases of lymphocytes, although neutrophils also decreased at Day 3 at 20 mg/kg. By Day 15, the lymphocytes were beginning to rebound at 10 and 15 mg/kg.

Treatment-related microscopic findings from necropsies (all animals) were limited to the bone marrow (femur, rib, and sternum), spleen, thymus, lymph nodes (mandibular and mesenteric), Peyer's patch, and sublingual salivary gland. Treatment-related depletions in the hematopoietic and lymphoid tissues were noted throughout the body. Bone marrow from of the femur, rib, and sternum had mild to moderate mixed depletion at 20 and 30 mg/kg. Mixed bone marrow depletion was characterized by decreased numbers of hematopoietic cells in erythroid, myeloid, lymphoid, and megakaryocytic lineages [16].

The spleen had minimal to moderate generalized lymphoid depletion in males at 10, 15, 20, and 30 mg/kg. Generalized lymphoid depletion in the thymus was considered to be increased in severity compared to controls in males at 15, 20, and 30 mg/kg. The mandibular and/or mesenteric lymph nodes had minimal to moderate generalized lymphoid depletion in males at 20 and 30 mg/kg. The Peyer's patch (gut-associated lymphoid tissue) had mild generalized lymphoid depletion in males at 20 and 30 mg/kg. Stress and/or an overall impairment of health potentially contributed to the development of hematopoietic and lymphoid depletion; however, these findings may indicate a direct test article effect in these animals. The sublingual salivary gland had minimal to moderate atrophy in males at 30 mg/kg. Salivary gland atrophy was potentially associated with a decrease in food intake; however, a direct test article-related effect cannot be ruled out [16]. The kidneys were normal [16].

The $LD_{10/50}$ for dogs was calculated to be 17.24/17.32 mg/kg. The experimental design is presented in **Tables 3** and **4**.

Study	Species and strain	No./sex	Age and wt	Route and mode	Pretest conditioning, dose and regimen	Results	Date/ laboratory
HOOI-12	Mice CD2F1	30 M 30 F	10 wks 19–24 g	IV Bolus	Single doses of 50–400 mg/kg of HOOI with observation × 15 days	LD_{10}—200 mg/kg	2007/ DEKK-TEC
793-017	Dogs Beagle	10 M	6 months 7.75–9.8 kg	IV Bolus	Single dose of 10–30 mg/kg of HOOI in a 24 day observation	LD_{10}—17.24 mg/kg LD_{50}—17.32 mg/kg	2008/MPI Research
Bevh-011	Hd Rats	20 F	10 wks 160–180 g	IP	Single doses of 100–150 mg/kg of HOOI and obs'd x 7 days	No evidence of impaired memory or learning	2008/ DEKK-TEC

Table 4. Acute toxicity summary study.

Table 4 summarizes the toxic effects of single IV dose administrations of HOOI in mice and dogs, which includes investigations on the acute toxicity performed in mice, rats, and dogs. The intravenous studies were conducted under FDA GLP guidelines [16].

4.3. Pharmacokinetics

The bioavailability for HOOI in one dog dosed once with IV HOOI 30 mg/kg is presented in **Figure 5**. The plasma HOOI was assayed employing the GC/MS method. In **Table 6**, all of the PK parameters are reviewed for all the dogs treated [16]. Overall, PK profile for HOOI in dogs revealed a two-compartment model with AUCs linear for all doses evaluated. The assay is sensitive to 20 ng/mL of HOOI [16]. Calculations were made as per methods previously reported [14, 15, 17, 21–23].

Model parameters were estimated using Micropharm software and nonlinear least squares regression was performed using Simplex and Gauss-Newton fitting algorithms (Statistical software available from Stat soft, Tulsa, OK) [17, 21]. An open two-compartment model provided the best fit. Clearance, volume of distribution, and half-lives were derived from estimates of the model parameters. Data analysis was performed on all plasma studies and analyzed via non-linear regression using a non-weighed quasi-Newtonian/simplex [17, 20, 21].

4.4. Brain/tumor penetration (CNS accumulation of drug)

Female athymic NCr-*nu*/*nu* mice were IC implanted with U25I glioma cells (10^6 cells) and divided into groups of 5 animals and administered HOOI (135 mg/kg/ day) in saline or saline (vehicle) (0.5 mL) IP daily for two consecutive days (qd × 2) beginning 4-day post inoculation

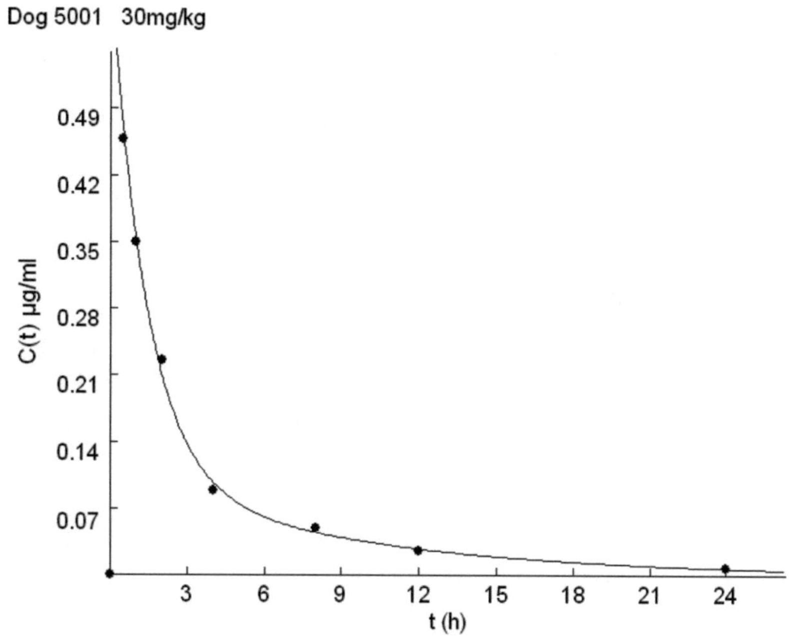

Figure 5. Bioavailability and pharmacokinetic profile for HOOI in dogs [16].

Parameter	15 mg/kg	20 mg/kg	30 mg/kg
AUC (mg·h/L)	0.49 0.39	0.96 1.49	1.66 1.14
Cl (L/h)	30.35 38.64	20.63 13.36	18.01 26.2
$T_{1/2}$ (h)	1.23 0.68	1.22 1.51	0.9 0.24
$T_{1/2}\beta$ (h)	3.19 3.09	15.6 13.56	6.05 1.85

Table 5. PK parameters in dogs treated with HOOI.

Drug	Species	Acute IV LD_{10}	Comparable human IV dosage*
HOOI	Mouse	200 mg/kg (600 mg/m^2)	60 mg/m^2 (10% of LD_{10})
HOOI	Dog	17.2 mg/kg (344 mg/m^2)	57 mg/m^2/d (1/6th of LD_{10})
*Standard conversion per FDA guidelines [26].			

Table 6. Estimated comparable human intravenous dosages*.

of cells. Four hours after the second treatment of each group, the animals were sacrificed and the brains removed intact and flash frozen in liquid nitrogen for storage [16, 17].

The encapsulated gliomas were easily identified and separated from normal brain with a scalpel and both homogenized separately in 10 mL 0.6 M phosphate buffer, pH 7.4 at 5°C [16, 17]. The cold homogenates were extracted with 10 mL chloroform, the organic layer separated and evaporated to dryness. HPLC and GC/MS analyses revealed HOOI in 100–126 ng/g glioma tissue. No drug was identified in the normal brain tissue homogenates. No chemicals or substances that could have interfered with the above extraction assays were noted in any of the tumors or normal brain tissues [16, 17].

4.5. Acute rat behavioral studies

HOOI vs. ifosfamide was evaluated in a modified rat neurobehavioral Morris water maze (18–20). Adult Sprague Dawley female rats (160–180 g) in groups of 3–6 rats per dosing were treated with single IP doses (MTD) of IFOS (400 mg/kg) vs. HOOI (200 mg/kg) vs. HOOI-Lys (300 mg/kg) and monitored with repeated timed swimming in the maze to find a hidden stage [17, 22–25].

The acute behavioral studies (latency to find a hidden platform in a Morris water maze—**Figures 6** and 7) was analyzed by variance (ANOVA) [17, 18].

Body weights and water temperature—prior to each dosing and during each assessment were monitored. Necropsies were performed on all rats [17].

There were no significant differences in behavior between the animals that received saline (controls), HOOI, and its lysine salt on the memory and learning time intervals. The IFOS-treated animals had shakes and tremors for >7 h. (secondary to chloroacetaldehyde), but demonstrated normal learning behavioral patterns. Five days later, all rats treated with IFOS demonstrated hemorrhagic cystitis with gross bleeding, and bone marrow evaluations revealed pancytopenia. HOOI- and the lysine salt-treated animals did reveal hemorrhagic cystitis, but renal tubular necrosis was not observed in any animals. Histological examinations confirmed the gross observations.

A control memory agent, MK-801, and 5-flurouracil (5-FU) were included to demonstrate complete and temporary impalement, respectively. Neither HOOI nor the lysine salt had any influence on memory or learning, in contrast to IFOS which produced long lasting impairment [8].

4.6. Plasma levels of 4-HOOI, chloroacetaldehyde and acrolein

Adult, female C3H mice were dosed with a single IV MTD of cyclophosphamide (CPA) (250 mg/kg), IFOS (400 mg/kg), or HOOI (100 mg/kg); dogs were dosed with IV HOOI (30 mg/kg). Blood was collected and measured for HOOI, chloroacetaldehyde, and acrolein.

IFOS released CAA and ACR during hepatic metabolism and GC/MS assays were employed to quantitate the plasma HOOI, CAA, and ACR generated. For ACR and CAA, the Kobayashi et al. procedure (involving a pentafluorophenylhydrazine derivatization) was modified, validated with pure CAA and ACR and biological samples [16, 21, 25].

http://dx.doi.org/10.5772/66304

HOOI did not generate any detectable plasma levels of CAA in mice, in contrast to IFOS [16]. There is a striking inefficiency in the metabolic activation of IFOS to IPM *in vivo* [supported in the observed IV single dose LD_{10} for HOOI vs. IFOS (200 vs. 470 mg/kg) in mice]. The highest tolerated single IV dose tolerated for IFOS was 400 mg/kg and for HOOI is 100 mg/kg. Ideally we would have liked to use HOOI at 400 mg/kg to equalize doses, but that would be too toxic for HOOI and to reduce IFOS would have made it too low [7, 8, 11, 16].

ACR plasma levels were lower for HOOI in both dogs and mice. Mice, rats, and dogs dosed with HOOI did not demonstrate urinary hemorrhagic cystitis, in contrast to the IFOS treated mice, in which hematuria occurred 5-days post dosing. The results support our hypothesis that subjects treated with HOOI vs. IFOS would be exposed to lower plasma levels of ACR and no CAA with potentially reduced risks of developing hemorrhagic cystitis and no neurotoxicity. This is in agreement with Carlson et al. who measured 2.12 μg/mL for CAA @ 4 h after 1-h infusion of IFOS (400 mg/kg) in a clinical study [10].

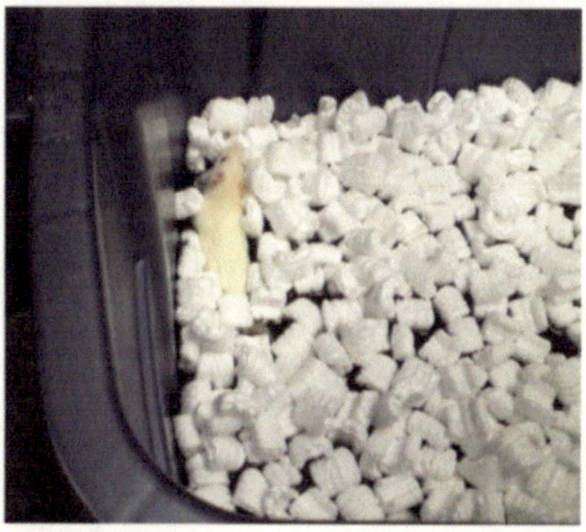

Figure 6. A rat swimming through the peanuts.

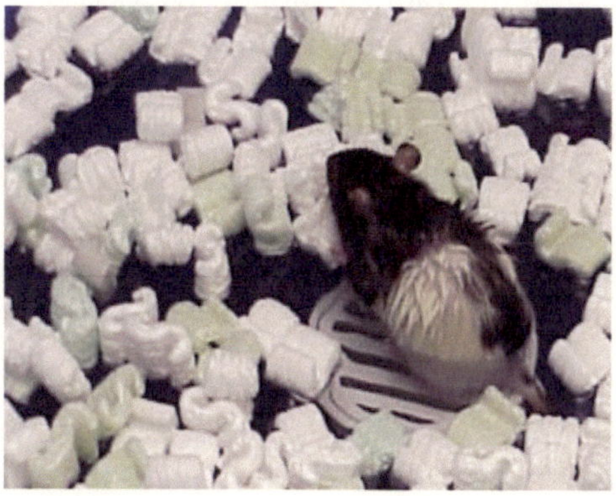

Figure 7. A rat on the hidden water maze platform.

5. Statistical analyses

Data analyses were performed on all plasma/tissue studies and analyzed with nonlinear regression methods using a nonweighed quasi-Newtonian/simplex fitting algorithms (Statistical software from Stat Soft, Tulsa, OK) [16, 17].

6. Discussion

The rationale for the preclinical development of HOOI was based on observed antitumor activity vs. intracranially implanted human tumor xenografts growing in mice and an anticipated reduction in renal toxicity and encephaloneuropathy that occur with standard IFOS and IPM therapy (1, 8, 9).

We review here the anticancer activities for HOOI in mice bearing intracranially implanted human xenografts and the results of acute toxicity and pharmacology studies with single intravenous injections in groups of mice and dogs. The end-point of all the studies was to document anticancer activity and drug toxicity for HOOI and an acceptable starting dose for a Phase I clinical trial in humans with advanced cancer. The anticancer activities, toxicology, and pharmacology studies reported in **Tables 1–4** support the clinical development of HOOI.

Human subjects treated with IFOS develop CNS toxicities which appear to be due to the CAA that is generated from the dechloroethylation of either of the two 2-chloroethyl moieties [2, 7, 10].

These cyclic mono-dechloroethylated metabolites of IFOS undergo 4-hydroxylation, resulting in a 4-hydroxyl dechloroethylated IFOS metabolite in which the ring opens resulting in the corresponding aldehydes with subsequent elimination of ACR. The use of HOOI would bypass the dechloroethylation step seen with IFOS. The ACR formation would be significantly reduced and therefore lead to a significant reduction in the incidence of hemorrhagic cystitis and renal tubular necrosis, which are common toxicities associated with IFOS therapy [2].

The observations presented in the **Table 5** support DEKK-TEC's hypothesis that subjects treated with HOOI vs. IFOS would be exposed to lower plasma levels of acrolein and no chloroacetaldehyde with potentially reduced risks of developing renal tubular necrosis and with no neurotoxicity. There is a striking inefficiency in the metabolic activation of IFOS to IPM *in vivo* (3). This is noted in the observed LD_{10} for HOOI vs. IFOS (200 vs. 470 mg/kg) in mice. Because of this, an effective clinical IFOS dose is harder to achieve because of intrasubject metabolism variability. Since HOOI does not require hepatic activation *in vivo*, a reduced intrasubject variability in the clinic is another potential advantage of administering HOOI.

Renal tubular necrosis and CNS toxicity have not been noted with HOOI in the animal studies. In the mouse study, HOOI did not generate any detectable chloroacetaldehyde and only 20% of the acrolein produced by equivalent doses of IFOS. The latter difference is because HOOI does not appear to be a substrate for microsomal metabolism and enters cancer cells intact and releases IPM and ACR *in situ*. Neither proximal tubular necrosis nor Fanconni syndrome was observed in the rat or dog studies at final necropsy [1–3, 11, 13].

http://dx.doi.org/10.5772/66304

Specific emphasis has been placed on documenting potential toxicities associated with IV administered HOOI, a peroxide—capable of producing convulsions, renal damage, hemolysis, arterial gas emboli-pulmonary damage, and neurological pathology—none of which have been noted.

In dog studies, animals that received HOOI, leukocytes, and neutrophils were moderately variable—decreased on Day 2 and at termination. Predominant organ(s) defect at autopsy was depletion of splenetic lymphocytes. Bone marrow was microscopically minimally to moderately depressed with acceptable ratios of blood elements. No other evidence of toxicity was noted at autopsies, including careful complete examinations of the bone marrow and brain.

All dogs in the 10 and 15 mg/kg dosage groups survived to the scheduled necropsy on Day 15, while groups administered 20 and 30 mg/kg were euthanized *in extremis* on Day 8 following veterinary consultation due to their deteriorating physical condition, primarily a worsening lack of appetite and associated/expected physical deterioration over time. At the gross necropsy of animals euthanized *in extremis*, three of the four animals had no findings while one animal exhibited mild red discoloration of the duodenum and mucosa of the small intestine. Other than spleens devoid of blood element precursors other pathology was noted.

Based on the results and outcomes of the dog HOOI study, the LD_{10} was calculated to be 17.2 mg/kg and the LD_{50} was 17.3 mg/kg. Thus, the intravenous LD_{10} single-dose value for mice and dogs (sexes combined) were calculated as 200 and 17.2 mg/kg, respectively, and agreed well.

Clinical studies have revealed very high urinary levels of ACR and CAA in subjects dosed with IFOS [10]. In one study, 48% of the dose was excreted as the dechloroethylated metabolites, while unchanged drug and carboxyifosfamide, the other major metabolite, accounted for only 4.7% and 2.2%, respectively [21]. Consequently, circulating levels of the dechloroethylated metabolites of IFOS could conceivably be a secondary source of CAA, in addition to the parent drug, which is very likely the primary source.

In the present study, the metabolism of HOOI *in vivo* was not observed to be a source of CAA. HOOI is probably less likely to be a substrate for cytochrome P450 oxidation to generate an exocyclic hemiacetal at an α-carbon in either of the two 2-chloroethyl moieties (with subsequent elimination of CAA), but is readily converted directly to carboxy-IFOS and IPM.

It is also reasonable to expect that clinical doses of HOOI would be significantly less than that for an equivalent amount of IFOS from the experimental studies (e.g., single MTD for HOOI 100 mg/kg vs. 400 mg/kg for IFOS), thus less drug would be available to form CAA. The bioavailability profile supports the single dose schedule, which is acceptable with the FDA [26].

HOOI possesses two (2) 3-high energy atom chains [**-OOH** and **-O-P->O**] (**Figure 1**), thus the drug more than enough 'fits' the criteria proposed earlier that high energy drugs like HOOI have a propensity to enter cancer cells- that are low in energy, but high in energy requirements [17]. Furthermore, the drug's lipophilicity and the ability to accumulate in glioblastomas growing in the brain, make it a very desirable drug to develop for the treatment of brain tumors [16, 17].

No CNS/behavioral alterations or toxicities have been noted for HOOI or its L-lysine salt [16, 19].

Thus, preclinical studies, conducted under GLP guidelines are reviewed and are supportive for HOOI's entry into Phase I clinical trials as treatment for advanced cancer with CNS involvement. **Table 6** reviews calculated starting doses, and data that satisfied the FDA's requirements for an IND [26]. The initial level of dosing in the Phase I clinical trial has been established as 60 mg/m^2 [9, 16, 19, 26].

7. Conclusion

Over all, the drug was well tolerated. Predictions for human pharmacokinetic parameters and dosing are made from allometric analyses using the above three species. Data predicted an acceptable starting dose of 60 mg/m^2 (from mouse and dog studies). The presented toxicity data plus strong antineuro-oncology activity supports HOOI's proposed use as treatment for CNS malignancies. The drug is being prepared for the US–IND pending Phase I trial studies [26].

Acknowledgement

Supported by the NCI/SBIR grants R43/44 CA094566.

Disclaimer

Multiple patents have been filed based on the information obtained for the drug, 4-hydroperoxyifosamaide (HOOI), from DEKK-TEC's group. Portions of that information plus techniques and results generated from our group that have been published are included in this chapter and appropriately referenced. All of the previously published studies and reports presented are referenced and are from DEKK-TEC's laboratories and contract facilities.

Author details

Lee Roy Morgan[1,*], Andrew H. Rodgers[1], Gerard Bastian[2], William S. Waud[3], Branko S. Jursic[2], Robert F. Struck[4], Gerald LaHoste[5] and Edward Stevens[2]

*Address all correspondence to: lrm1579@aol.com

1 DEKK-TEC, Inc., New Orleans, LA, USA

2 Department of Chemistry, University of New Orleans, Lakefront, New Orleans, LA, USA

3 Southern Research Institute, Birmingham, AL, USA

4 Cancermedica, LLC, Birmingham, AL, USA

5 Department of Psychology, University of New Orleans, Lakefront, New Orleans, LA, USA

References

[1] Struck, RF, Dykes, DJ, Corbett, TH, Suling, WJ and Trader, MW. Isophosphoroamide mustard, a metabolite of ifosfamide with activity against murine tumors comparable to cyclophosphamide. Br. J. Cancer. 47:15–26, 1983.

[2] Norpoth, K. Studies on the metabolism of isophosphamide in man. Cancer Treat. Rep. 60:437–443, 1976.

[3] Gale, RP, van Vugt, A, Rosen, L, Struck, RF, Morgan, LR and LoRusso, P. ZIO-201: A Phase 1 study of isophosphoramide mustard (IPM-lysine) in advanced cancers. ASCO. 24:524, 2006.

[4] Gale, RP, Morgan, LR, Struck, RF, Rosen, L and LoRusso, P. Use of isophosphoramide mustard lysine (ZIO-201) as therapy for lymphoma. Int. Soc. Hematology. 17:21, 2006.

[5] Germain, R, Bastian, G., Serota, D, Struck, RF and Morgan, LR. Isophosphophamide mustard (IPM): Preclinical pharmacology and toxicology in rodents, dogs and primates. Cancer Chemother. Pharmacol. 51: 1204–1212, 2004.

[6] Zolwyski, M and Baker, LH. Ifosfamide. J. Natl. Cancer Inst. 80:556–566, 1988.

[7] Goren, MP, Wright, RK, Pratt, CB and Pell, FE. Dechloroethylation of ifosfamide and neurotoxicity. Lancet. 2:1219–1220, 1986.

[8] Morgan, L.R, Struck, RF, Rodgers, AH, Jursic, BS and Waud, WR. Pre-clinical pharmacology and toxicology for 4-hydeoperoxyifosfamide (HOOI) and its L-lysine Salt – A novel anticancer agent. Am. Assoc Cancer Res. 42: 3222, 2011.

[9] Morgan, LR, Struck, RF, Rodgers, AH, Jursic, BS, Waud, WS and Butera, D. Development of Clinical Products. NCI Translational Science Meeting, Washington, DC, 2008.

[10] Carlson, L, Goren, MP, Bush, DA, Griener, JC, Quigley, R, Tkaczewski, I, Kamen, BA and Weitman, SD. Toxicity, pharmacokinetics, and in vitro hemodialysis clearance of ifosfamide and metabolites in an anephric pediatric patient with Wilm's tumor. Cancer Chemother. Pharmacol. 41:140–146, 1998.

[11] Cox, PJ. Cyclophosphamide cystitis – Identification of acrolein as the causative agent. Biochem. Pharmacol. 28:2045–2049, 1979.

[12] Struck, RF, McCain, DM, Tendian, SW and Tillery, KH. Quantification of 4-hydroxyifosfamide in plasma of ifosfamide-treated mice. Cancer Chemother. Pharmacol. 40:57–59, 1997.

[13] Takamizawa, A, Iwata, T, Yamaguchi, K, Shiratori, O, Harada, M, Tochino, Y and Matsumoto, S. Stereochemistry, metabolism and antitumor activity of 4-hydroperoxy-isophosphamide and its stereoisomer. Cancer Treat. Rep. 60:361–368, 1976.

[14] Hohorst, HJ, Peter, G and Struck, RF. Synthesis of 4-hydroperoxy derivatives of ifosfamide and trofosfamide by direct ozonation and preliminary antitumor evaluation in vivo. Cancer Res. 36:2278–2281, 1976.

[15] Takamizawa, A, Matsumoto, S, Iwata, T and Makino, I. Synthesis, stereochemistry and antitumor activity of hydroperoxy isophosphoramide and related compounds. Chem. Pharm. Bull. (Japan) 25:1877–1888, 1977.

[16] Morgan, LR. Complexes of 4-hydroperoxyifosfamide as anti-tumor agents. US Patent 8,361,992, 2013 and worldwide patents.

[17] Morgan, LR, Rodgers, AH, Bastian, G, Benes, E, Waud, WR, Jursic, BS, Struck, RF, LaHoste, G, Thornton, M, Luttrell, M, Stevens, E and Thompson, R. Comparative preclinical pharmacology and toxicology for 4-demethyl-4-cholestryloxycarbonylpenclomedine (DM-CHOC-PEN): A potential neuro-alkylating agent for glioblastoma and metastatic cancers of the central nervous system. *In*: CNS Tumors, Ed. Lee Roy Morgan, InTech Publishing, Croatia, 2014.

[18] Morgan, L.R., Struck, R.F., Rodgers, A.H., Jursic, B.S. Waud, W.R. Carbonate and carbamate derivatives of 4-demethylpenclomedine as novel anticancer agents. Cancer Chemother. Pharmacol. 64: 829–835, 2009.

[19] Morgan, LR, A rational for novel anti-neurooncology drugs. Chapter 15. *In*: Evolution of the Molecular Biology of Brain Tumors and The Therapeutic Implications, Ed. Terry Lichtor, InTech Publishing, Croatia, 435–458, 2013.

[20] Chiou, WL. Critical evaluation of the potential error in pharmacokinetic studies of using linear trapezoidal rule method for the calculation of the area under the plasma level-time curve. J. Pharmacokinet Biopharm. 6:539–546, 1978.

[21] Dupont, MK. The estimate of moments: A technical note. J. Pharmacokinet Biopharm. 17: 203–208, 1989.

[22] Morris, R. Development of water-maze procedure for studying spatial learning in the rat. J. Neurosci. Methods. 11:47–60, 1984.

[23] Morgan, LR, Thornton, ME, Benes, EN, Struck, RF, Jursic, BS, Rodgers, RH, Bastian, G, LaHoste, G and Thompson, RB. Neurobehavioral properties of penclomedine (PEN) and other agents. EORTC, Molecular Targets and Therapeutics, Geneva, 2008.

[24] Saab, BJ, Saab, AMP and Roder, JC. Statistical and theoretical considerations for the platform re-location water maze. J. Neurosci. Methods. 198:44–52, 2011.

[25] Kobayashi, K, Tanaka, M and Kawai, S. Gas chromatographic determination of low molecular weight carbonyl compounds in aqueous solutions as their O-(2,3,4,5,6-pentafluorobenzyl) oximes. J. Chromatogr. 187:413–415, 1980.

[26] Morgan, LR. Discussions with the US FDA regarding an IND for 4-hydroperoxyifosfamide, Feb. 6, 2016.